Post-Baby Bounce

Namita Jain's illustrious career in the wellness space spans more than twenty-five years. Today, she is highly regarded as a wellness specialist. Over the years, Namita has continuously stayed ahead of the curve by remaining on top of new trends and techniques in her field. She stands out from the rest, equipped as she is with an unmatched list of qualifications and prestigious international certifications in numerous health-related disciplines:

American Council of Exercise:
- Lifestyle and Weight Management Consultant
- Clinical Exercise Specialist
- Group Training Specialist

American College of Sports Medicine:
- Health and Fitness Instructor

Aerobic and Fitness Association of America:
- Group Health Instructor (Aerobics and Step)

Pilates UK Institute:
- Pilates Master Trainer

Namita is a contributing writer on nutrition, fitness and various health-related issues for numerous leading newspapers and magazines. She has authored several books and her best-sellers include:
- *Jaldi Fit with Namita Jain* (with DVD): *A Complete Workout Guide for Adults*
- *Jaldi Fit Kids with Namita Jain: Ten Food and Fitness Mantras for Children*
- *The Four-*___ *Diet: A Diet and Lifestyle Guide*
- *Figure*___ *ess*

- *Sexy @ Sixty: Health and Beauty at Every Age*
- *How to Lose the Last 5 Kilos: And Feel on Top of the World*
- *Fit Pregnancy: The Complete Health Plan for You and Your Baby*
- *Jaldi Fit A to Z: The Complete Wellness Guide*
- *9 to 5 Fit: A Working Person's Guide to Looking Great and Performing Better*

In the field of rehabilitation, Namita offers consultations at Bombay Hospital as a clinical wellness specialist. Here she conducts one-on-one as well as group sessions on diet, exercise, lifestyle and weight management.

Her association with Diet Mantra is a pan-Indian venture where she trains dieticians in the art of healthy eating for a healthy life; its aim is weight loss with a purpose. Namita Jain was also the nutrition partner for Femina Miss India 2012. She features as a nutritionist on the TV channel Food Food in the health cookery programme *Health Maange More.*

Despite her busy schedule, Namita continues to hold classes in aerobics, yoga, Pilates, step workout and interval training. Her company, Live Active, and her brand, Jaldi Fit, have rapidly become household names in health and lifestyle products and services.

For more information on Namita Jain and her wellness programmes, log on to her websites, www.liveactive.com and www.jaldifit.com.

Post-Baby Bounce

NAMITA JAIN

Collins

First published in India in 2015 by Collins
An imprint of HarperCollins *Publishers*

P-ISBN: 978-93-5136-488-7
E-ISBN: 978-93-5136-489-4

2 4 6 8 10 9 7 5 3 1

HarperCollins *Publishers*
A-75, Sector 57, Noida, Uttar Pradesh – 201301, India
77-85 Fulham Palace Road, London W6 8JB, United Kingdom
Hazelton Lanes, 55 Avenue Road, Suite 2900, Toronto, Ontario M5R 3L2
and 1995 Markham Road, Scarborough, Ontario M1B 5M8, Canada
25 Ryde Road, Pymble, Sydney, NSW 2073, Australia
195 Broadway, New York, NY 10007, USA

Typeset in 10/14 Mercury Display by
Jojy Philip, New Delhi 110 015

Printed and bound at
Thomson Press (India) Ltd

Contents

Preface

Losing weight, even in normal circumstances, is a difficult proposition. And when you have just delivered and have a baby to look after, it becomes even more challenging. That is what gave me the idea for this book.

Motherhood—such a cocktail of emotions! One moment, you are on top of the world. The next, you find yourself hurtling through a thunderstorm of uncertainty and panic. No matter how much you've looked forward to being a mother, there will always be moments when you feel you aren't sufficiently prepared for the responsibility. Many new mothers like you find yourself caught in a dilemma. On the one hand, you want to spend every waking moment with the baby. On the other, you are already thinking up ways to return to work or itching to hit the gym to get back your lost figure. *Post-Baby Bounce* understands your dilemma and promises to help you resolve it, to your satisfaction, by suggesting ways in which you can devote time to yourself without feeling as if you are cheating on your baby.

For all practical purposes, weight loss is governed by two heavily publicized core factors—diet and exercise. And while they may seem deceptively simple, only a new mother like you knows that it isn't so! There are many factors that will try to undermine your commitment to them. And that's what makes this book different from other weight-loss guides. It attempts to initiate a dialogue with you, the new mother, tries to understand the predicaments that are unique to your situation and offers the best solutions possible within a given framework.

Trust me, there is nothing selfish or wrong about wanting to feel and look good. Only make sure that you take it slow and steady. I want you, as a reader, to take this one lesson away from the book: No matter how impossible a situation may seem, everything is possible as long as you put your heart into it.

SECTION ONE

JUST DELIVERED

'Suddenly she was here. And I was no
longer pregnant; I was a mother. I never
believed in miracles before.'
— Ellen Greene, American actress

In the course of my career, I've encountered many new mothers, each one different from the next. Some women expect miracles from me—miracles that would have them walking the ramp for Victoria's Secret a mere month after giving birth. Others are reluctant to follow any kind of regimen and have to be mollycoddled and coaxed into sparing some me-time. These mothers aren't happy about their weight but they lack the motivation to do something about it. Some of them believe that they can merely exercise their way to a slim figure. Others feel that they only need to diet to regain their previous selves. Regardless of what course of action they decide to take, they all have one thing in common—they want instant dramatic results.

However, the one thing they forget is that they do not have Superwoman's body. No matter what kind of delivery they've had—normal or Caesarean—they would have to allow some time for rest and recovery. Only afterwards should they try to get into any kind of regimen. To make them understand the reason, I have attempted in this section to explain just what delivering a child means to a woman's body. Once they know the extent of the changes that have taken place within them will they realize why it is important to bide their time.

1
Normal vs Caesarean Delivery

Dear Diary,

I haven't written in a while, I know, and you must be dying to hear the latest. I am a mom! Of a healthy baby girl. Ten toes. Ten fingers. And the most adorable crinkly smile ever. She's perfect. It certainly wasn't easy, though, and while I had had my heart set on a normal delivery, doctors decided that a C-section would be best for both the baby and me. I am still in the hospital, still a little exhausted by the ordeal, still slightly dopey, thanks to all the medication ... but as I stare at the tiny bundle in my arms, it seems to have been worth it.

For now,
S.

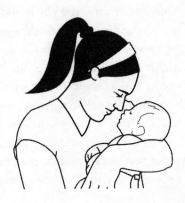

Normal delivery

Normal delivery means giving birth through the vaginal opening. Usually, with every push, the tissues stretch wide enough for the baby to slide through. Sometimes, though, there may be vaginal tears involving the skin around the vagina caused by the baby coming out, or the doctor may consider an episiotomy to ensure that the opening is large enough for the delivery.

What you need to know:

Recovery time after a normal delivery depends on whether there were any complications. Both vaginal tearing and episiotomy require stitches; they will hurt for a while and lengthen the recovery period for new mothers.

How to deal with the discomfort after returning home:

✓ Apply ice packs to the affected area to take the edge off the pain.
✓ Practise good hygiene to avoid infection.
✓ To ease pressure, sit down on a soft cushion.
✓ Practise the Kegel exercises. Lie down on your back, bend your knees, gently tilt or raise the pelvis and squeeze the muscles as if to stop the flow of urine. Make sure you aren't contracting the muscles in your stomach as you do this. If you do it right, the perineum—the skin-covered area between the vagina and anus—will contract. Many women have difficulty locating the pelvic muscles, so try it in front of a mirror first and, with practice, you will be able to master the technique. Using the wrong muscles—such as your abs—won't give you the necessary benefits. Hold for five to ten seconds, then release. Try to do three to four sets of 25

repetitions several times throughout the day. In the second variation, perform ten rapid contractions and releases, several times a day. This will strengthen the muscles in your pelvic region.

✓ Wait until the stitches dissolve or are taken out, and then start gentle exercises, such as stretching and walking.

Caesarean delivery

Also called the C-section, it involves surgically removing the baby from the mother's uterus. The doctor may recommend it if he considers it vital for either the mother's or the baby's health. This is major surgery and requires an abdominal incision under anaesthesia; it is usually conducted as close to the due date as possible or about a week or two before, and it takes the mother a much longer time for recovery. For Srishti, it took her nearly six weeks to regain her energy and to overcome the constant feeling of exhaustion which followed her C-section.

What you need to know:

✓ The external incision itself may heal in a fortnight, but the uterus will take longer, usually six weeks, to recover.

✓ Like any other wound, this one is likely to hurt. Don't hesitate to ask your doctor for painkillers if you find the pain unbearable.

✓ It is all right to feel exhausted; it is only to be expected after a major procedure.

✓ If your stitches aren't the dissolving kind, you may be asked to return in a week's time to have them taken out.

✓ Sneezing and coughing may cause pain. The simplest of actions—sitting, standing, walking—will feel like a chore.

✓ Post-operation, the intestines tend to be sluggish and can cause a build-up of gas.

✓ Immediately after delivery, clearing your bowels can be an issue. The sooner you are allowed to take in solid food, the quicker you can put that in order.

✓ In the first few weeks, backache is quite common; pregnancy isn't easy on your back and it needs time to bounce back to normal.

✓ Incontinence due to stress or loss of bladder control is a possibility.

How to deal with it:

✓ Gentle stretching exercises to improve your circulation will help to make moving about a bit easier. To begin with, try walking, stretching your legs, flexing your toes, and moving from side to side. Ask your doctor to recommend some easy moves for you.

✓ Avoid heavy meals. Light, gas-dispelling foods, coupled with the above exercises, will ease the build-up of gas.

✓ To protect yourself from involuntary urination, use panty liners. The Kegel exercises will help you regain control of your bladder. Drink eight to ten glasses of water a day.

2

Changes in the Body

Dear Diary,

I am home now but I still feel a little sore from the delivery. Sore and overwhelmed. To be honest, I was so caught up with being pregnant that I never envisioned a time when the baby would be out and I would be faced with new situations which I wouldn't know how to handle. Just the physical changes are freaking me out. I'd heard about tender breasts and sagging tummy, sure, but who knew having a baby could affect simple things, such as sitting down, peeing and even bowel movements. I am losing hair too. Lots of it! Am I up to my new role as a mother? God, I don't know.

Panic-stricken,
S.

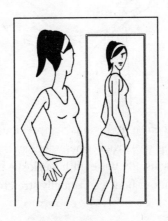

Srishti admits that she was aware of the changes which her body would go through during pregnancy but she was completely unprepared for what was to follow. It was only to be expected that it would take time and exercise for her stomach to get back into shape or that lactation would make her breasts feel heavy and even a little sore, but inability even to sit down? Loss of bladder control which would continue for more than just a couple of months? Hair loss? She wishes she had known better and had been better prepared to handle all these changes. Given her delicate hormonal state, these variables were more than enough to trigger occasional panic attacks.

As most women who have gone through it will tell you, motherhood is a sweet blessing but it does have its side effects, some of which linger on after delivery. In my experience, the more you know about them beforehand the easier it will be to manage them.

Flabby tummy

Pregnancy stretches your stomach to its limits and it will

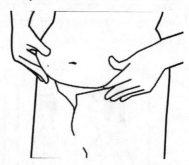

be some time before it regains its previous shape. Srishti remembers being awestruck when she saw her friend Divya pregnant with twins: 'By her eighth week she had grown huge. It's a miracle that our body can actually stretch that much,' she says in surprise.

Duration: It depends on how consistently and sincerely you exercise, but you should be able to get good results in a year's time.

How to deal with it: There is only one thing to do—exercise, exercise, exercise, but slowly and steadily. (Please read exercise section.)

Vaginal bleeding

This is usually no cause for worry—it is only your body cleaning up after delivery, ejecting leftover tissue and blood from the uterus. The flow will vary for different women.

Duration: This may last from a few weeks to about three months.

How to deal with it: It may be heavier than your usual period, but is easily taken care of with sanitary pads. Consider consulting a doctor only if it gets too profuse, is malodorous and is accompanied by fever.

Sore breasts

A build-up of milk production can make your breasts feel heavy and uncomfortable. Dryness or infection around the nipples is also possible. Also, as Srishti says, 'Having a kid latch on to your breast feels uncomfortable in the beginning and it took me some time to get used to it.'

Duration: Sore breasts usually develop a few days after delivery. They will occur only if the mother has not fed the baby frequently or not expressed the milk out.

How to deal with it: Frequent nursing to avoid build-up should do the trick. If not, try to relieve the discomfort with a hot water bottle and a massage. To avoid infection keep the area clean and moisturize it with milk cream.

Perineum woes

Pain in the vaginal area makes sitting down for long periods
uncomfortable, especially if you've had an episiotomy.

Duration: It usually takes about six weeks for the episiotomy
wound to heal and the vaginal area to strengthen.

How to deal with it: Take frequent breaks and lie down,
preferably on one side, to ease the pressure. If you *must* sit,
place a soft cushion or rubber ring underneath. Bathing the area
in warm water will bring relief. If there is any swelling, your
doctor might recommend ice packs. In addition, keep practising
the Kegel exercises. These will help strengthen your abdominal
muscles as well. If clearing your bowels is particularly painful,
you may consult your doctor about using painkillers.

Hair loss, dry skin

During pregnancy, the extra burst of hormones makes your
hair look lush. By that same principle, a post-pregnancy drop in
hormonal level leads to hair loss. It is only a temporary phase—
though a cause for much heartache—and your hair will go back
to its pre-pregnancy state soon enough. The same hormonal
changes may also give you dry skin.

Duration: About six months.

How to deal with it: Avoid excessive hair styling during this
time. If your doctor permits, you could take some supplements
to prevent excessive hair fall. For dry skin, drink lots of water
and be generous with the moisturizer.

Reservations about sex

It is best to wait out the recovery period before resuming sexual
relations. In that time, your body will heal itself and regain its
energy. For most new mothers, fatigue is also a pressing issue.

Keeping up with the baby's demands and the odd hours can crowd out sex.

> **Duration**: Wait for four to six weeks to reduce risk of infection, bleeding or reopening of stitches.
>
> **How to deal with it**: If soreness in the vaginal area continues to be a problem, experiment with different positions which do not put undue pressure on it. Communicate your feelings with your partner; let him know if something causes you pain. There might be some dryness in the vagina, in which case you can consult your doctor about the right lubrication to ease things. It is okay to be tired and to say so, but your relationship will benefit from spending quality time with your partner when the baby is asleep.

Swollen feet

They are caused by water retention and will improve with regular urination.

> **Duration**: Not more than one or two weeks.
>
> **How to deal with it**: Drink the recommended eight to ten glasses of water a day. Gentle exercises, such as walking and flexing or rotating your ankles will benefit you.

Cramps

They are usually a sign that your uterus is shrinking back to its normal size. They help prevent excessive bleeding by pressing down on the blood vessels. The more pregnancies you've undergone, the more severe the cramps are likely to be, possibly because multiple births affect muscle tone through constant stretching and shrinking.

> **Duration**: Not more than a week. If they last longer, consult your doctor.

Exhaustion

Dancing to your baby's tunes isn't easy. The work is demanding and there are no fixed hours. Often, just when you think the baby is asleep and you can put your feet up and finally have a short rest, it is time to get up and start the cycle all over again. Coming close on the heels of the delivery—which in itself is a painful and laborious process—it is no wonder that new mothers often complain of exhaustion. As long as it is just tiredness, it is all right. If you start falling into fits of depression and if you feel continuously lethargic and disinterested, you should seek the help of a doctor.

Duration: It could last through the breast feeding period, though this will vary from mother to mother.

How to deal with it: Turn on your charm and get your family to help with the household chores. They can also babysit while you grab that much-needed shut-eye. Let your baby be your priority and stop stressing about the dust on the furniture, the laundry on the living-room floor, and so on. Put that cell phone to good use and order home delivery of groceries and other essentials, in bulk if necessary so they don't have to be replenished too often. It is okay to order takeaways if you don't have time to cook, but ensure that your choices are healthy. Salads, piping hot soups, idlis, dal-khichdi are ideal, as are milkshakes and smoothies. Keep fruits like bananas handy for instant energy. Energy bars, digestive biscuits and yoghurt make great snacks. Make sure you drink plenty of water too.

Constipation

The first bowel movement after delivery comes with its own baggage. The strain of delivering a baby affects the abdominal muscles—as well as another condition called diastasis recti(see glossary for details)—the bowels and, by extension, the process of elimination. A new mother's anticipation of pain or fear of the stitches splitting may also trigger constipation.

Duration: It will depend on your lifestyle but, again, the experience will differ from mother to mother.

How to deal with it: A good diet will help ease the process of elimination. Make sure your food packs a lot of fibre in the form of fresh fruits, vegetables, wholegrains, pulses and sprouts. Prunes are particularly effective in dealing with constipation. Drink lots of water as well. Start your day with warm water and lemon juice. Simple exercises, such as walking and gentle stretches, will aid digestion and prevent bowel troubles. If you get no relief, ask your doctor about using laxatives. A topical anaesthetic gel may help ease the pain.

Piles

The strains and stresses of pregnancy and constipation can lead to haemorrhoids or piles and cause bleeding during elimination.

Duration: It will vary from mother to mother although problems may persist even after breastfeeding comes to an end.

How to deal with it: If you are suffering from constipation, deal with it first. Drink lots of water to soften stool and enable them to move out. If the condition persists, consult your doctor.

Peeing troubles

Most new mothers don't feel an urge to urinate for the first day or two. And if they do, they may find the flow unsatisfactory, irregular or accompanied by some pain. There could be many reasons for that. One, the bladder gets stretched during pregnancy in order to hold more fluid. Second, it may be a reflex action generated to avoid pain in the vaginal area. Third, if you have stitches, the wound may cause a burning sensation when you are passing urine. Finally, if you are confined to bed and have to use a bed pan, sheer embarrassment may prevent you from peeing.

Duration: Not more than a day or two.

How to deal with it: Even if you don't feel like it, try and empty your bladder every six to eight hours. Drink lots of water and walk around a bit to ease it. Consult your doctor if it feels full despite frequent urination.

Stress incontinence

Incontinence is the inability to hold urine back because of weakness in the pelvic muscles which support the bladder. The shrinking of the uterus after delivery also puts extra pressure on the bladder, making it difficult to hold back the flow, especially when you cough, sneeze or laugh hard.

Duration: About three to six months.

How to deal with it: As mentioned under Caesarean delivery, drink lots of water and practise the Kegel exercises. Urinate frequently at first, gradually increasing the time between your visits to the loo.

Backache

As your stomach expands during the last few months of pregnancy, your back takes a beating. It will be some time before its ligaments regain their strength and snap back into shape.

Duration: It may be several weeks before this problem gets off your back.

How to deal with it: Gentle exercise is what your back needs. If the pain gets unmanageable, get your doctor to prescribe something for it.

Take it from me: It is easy to fret over the possible after-effects of delivering a baby, but remember that they will last only a little while. More importantly, this post-partum phase will speed past at a gallop and then, try as you might, you won't be able to turn back the clock. So why not make the most of it? Forget everything else. Just relax, breathe deeply and savour every moment that you spend with your newborn. It will be good for the baby and for your body. One year down the line, all you will remember of this phase is what brought you the most joy: your baby's wondrous, trusting smile, his bubbling laughter and his many accomplishments—crawling, walking, talking. Everything you've gone through will feel totally worth it. I leave you with a wonderful entry from Srishti's diary:

Dear Diary,

The moments of self-doubt have come and gone (though I am sure they will keep making guest appearances for the next twenty-odd years at least!). It is very soothing to see Mia (yes, that's what I call her secretly though nobody knows that yet) sound asleep by my side. It is like she already trusts my presence. It's fun to observe her—the tiny, balled-up fists, the occasional gaping yawn, the closed eyes moving under her almost-translucent lids as if dreaming a small dream—and it is difficult not to get all choked up. Yes, God is in his heaven and all is right with my world. Good night,

S.

Glossary of Terms	
Caesarean	It may have come from the Latin 'caedere', meaning 'to cut'. It involves making an incision just above the pubic bone first and then into the uterus to remove the baby. It is usually performed under anaesthesia—spinal, epidural or general.
Diastasis recti	This is a condition in which your abdominal muscles get separated during the trauma of giving birth, leaving a ridge down the middle of your abdomen. You can feel this space when

	you are lying on your back. Inform your doctor and he will recommend special exercises for it.
Engorged breasts	They are so called when there is an excessive build-up of milk in your breasts.
Episiotomy	It is a surgical procedure that involves making an incision in a way that enlarges the vaginal opening to allow the baby to slide out easily. It is performed under local anaesthesia.
Haemorrhoids, Piles	It refers to dilation of the veins of the anus or the rectum, in this case due to childbirth. It can cause pain, itchiness and bleeding.
Lochia	The medical term for vaginal bleeding after delivery.

BREASTFEEDING AND LACTATION

More and more mothers are actively endorsing exclusive breastfeeding for the first six months, and rightly so. No formula milk can ever duplicate the benefits of breast milk which is packed with just the nutrients which your baby needs after birth. Not only is it nourishing in terms of lactose, fat and calorie content but it also provides the baby with the adequate health insurance cover that will go a long way in his growth and development. Breast milk is said to be packed with antibodies that boost immunity against infections; it improves digestion by promoting healthy bacteria in the baby's stomach. It is even believed to protect your child from various conditions, such as allergies, asthma, eczema and tooth cavities. Breastfeeding is a way of spending quality time with your baby and I believe that it helps recreate some of that closeness you felt when the baby was still in the womb.

As a new mother, you too can benefit a lot from it. It hastens the recovery process after delivery by lowering the risk of bleeding and by speeding up the contraction of the enlarged uterus. It also helps you regain your pre-pregnancy figure faster by utilizing the extra fat in milk production (yes, you heard that right!). In most cases, breastfeeding can be a calming influence on both the mother and the child.

As with all new experiences, breastfeeding can be daunting at first but you will find yourself easing into this routine after only a few tries. This section will give you enough tips and tricks to make this a comfortable time for both you and the baby. And since many new mothers are often in the dark about diet and exercise in the lactating and breastfeeding phase, I have laid down a few ground rules that you can follow.

3

Nursing Your Baby

Dear Diary,

Right from the beginning, breastfeeding hasn't been the pain I had expected it to be. At first, it was uncomfortable but I got used to it pretty quickly. Mia demands to be fed regularly but doesn't create too much fuss while at it and seems content and at ease later. My friend who bore twins didn't have such an easy time. Having two mouths to feed meant she was nursing all the time and it was tiring (she did try feeding them simultaneously but didn't enjoy the process any better). It made her and, in turn, her babies, quite cranky. It is things like these that make me realize how blessed I am.

S.

Based on my experiences, I can tell you that every mother will have a different story to tell and while Srishti was lucky enough with the nursing, others may not be quite as fortunate and may end up feeling tense and anxious about it. Especially those who, like Srishti's friend, are dealing with a multiple birth. Patience can be your best friend at such times. If you are calm and patient, it is likely that the baby will be too. And if you are having trouble, why not enlist the help of your mother and other women in your family? They will have enough anecdotes and handy hints to ensure you don't run out of ideas even when you are at the end of your tether.

What you need to know:

✓   The stimulus for milk production is suckling. Suckling triggers the release of the hormones prolactin and oxytocin which are required for milk production.

✓   The breasts produce colostrum, a milky fluid packed with nutrients. Along with other health benefits, it assists in the moving of meconium or stool out of the baby's body.

✓   Newborns usually nurse eight to twelve times a day for the first few weeks. Later, they will need to feed about six to eight times a day.

✓   Stress can hinder the release of milk while nursing. It is also possible that the mother's mood may pass on to the baby and spoil matters further.

How to deal with it:

✓   Choose a comfortable spot to nurse, one that is cool, quiet and without distractions.

✓   Put your legs up, use pillows and generally make yourself comfortable.

✓   Play some calming music to improve your mood.

✓   Do some relaxation exercises:

   i.   Deep breathing (to be repeated five times):

         Sit up straight and breathe slowly. As you breathe in, breathe in calmness. As you breathe out, breathe out tension and anxiety.

   ii.   Shoulder rolls (to be repeated three times forward and three times back):

         With arms hanging loosely by your side, rotate your

shoulders from front to back. Inhale while your shoulders go up and back; exhale while they come down and in front. Then rotate shoulders from back to front.

iii. Neck movements (to be repeated six times on each side):

Turn your head to the right, inhaling as you turn and exhaling as you return to position.

Repeat on the left in the same manner.

✓ Feeding may take time, so keep water and some snacks handy to replenish yourself.

✓ Lactation specialists have come up with different positions for breastfeeding. These are:

i. Crossover hold

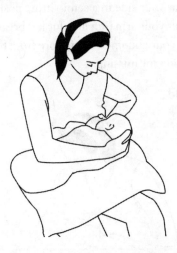

If you are nursing on the left breast, hold your baby with the right hand, and vice versa. Provide adequate support to your baby's head by holding him between the shoulder blades, the thumb behind one ear and the fingers behind the other.

ii. Football hold

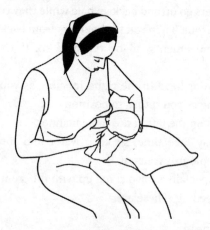

Place the baby at your side in a semi-sitting position; the baby's legs will be under your arm (left arm for left breast, right arm for right breast). If your abdomen is still sore from the delivery, this is a better position for nursing.

iii. Cradle hold

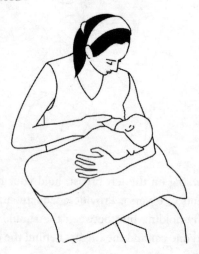

Here, the baby's head rests in the crook of your arm. This is for when you become more comfortable with nursing.

iv. Sideways hold

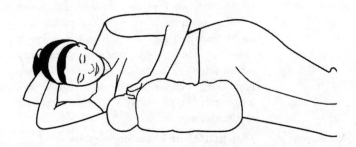

Here, both of you lie down on your sides, tummy to tummy; ideal for middle-of-the-night nursing.

v. Simultaneous feeding

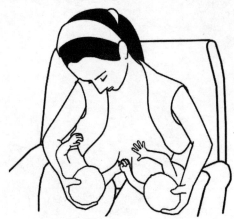

If you have twins, try nursing them simultaneously. Use the football hold for both babies or combine the football and the cradle holds. Use oversized nursing pillows to ensure their heads are well supported.

Glossary of Terms	
Colostrum	In the first two days after delivery, the breasts produce colostrum, a yellowish fluid packed with antibodies which have antivirus and antibacterial properties which boost your baby's immunity against infections. It contains enzymes which help improve digestion, and proteins which regulate iron. It also acts as a mild laxative which enables the baby to pass his first stool.
Meconium	The scientific term for the baby's first stool.
Prolactin	The hormone which stimulates milk production.
Oxytocin	The hormone which directs milk flow through the ducts. Both prolactin and oxytocin are secreted in the brain.

4

Nutrition and Breastfeeding

Dear Diary,

There is so much to occupy my mind these days that I haven't really been paying attention to what I am eating. My meals are healthy enough, I think, but all the in-betweens will qualify as nothing but junk. And to top it all, I had a little wine last night. I felt I deserved it after months of abstention. I know my doctor wouldn't approve but eating seems too trivial a thing to worry about now.

S.

Srishti may have thought food a very trivial matter in the face of so many other things that she was experiencing, and she said as much when she approached me. But, trust me, it is not— not only because it is not doing your health any good but also because, just like during your pregnancy, you aren't eating only for yourself, you are eating for your baby as well. As such, your diet should, qualitatively and quantitatively, fulfil your own and your baby's nutritive requirements. You must understand that what you eat is what will eventually end up in your baby's tummy via breast milk. So I would advise you to consider your food choices wisely. To make monitoring easy, write down what you are eating. It will put things in perspective for you and keep you from indulging yourself too often, and too unwisely.

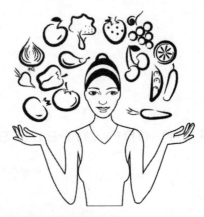

What you need to know:

✓   Studies suggest that while you are breastfeeding you need an additional 550 calories during the first six months and an extra 400 calories in the subsequent six months after your delivery.

✓   Both coffee and chocolate contain stimulants (caffeine and the obromide respectively). They are difficult to metabolize and can make your baby restless.

✓   Does any member of your family have any food allergy? It is possible your kid has inherited it.

✓   Drugs have a way of getting absorbed into breast milk and their effects can transfer into the baby as well.

✓   Milk production gets reduced if the water intake is inadequate, that is, less than two to three litres a day.

How to deal with it:

✓   Restrict coffee intake to two cups or less per day. Consume chocolate sparingly.

✓   Even if you are now allowed alcohol, restrict drinking to not more than two glasses a week. To ensure that the alcohol has cleared from your bloodstream, it is better to nurse your child before you drink, or to delay it till a few hours afterwards.

✓ Even if you do not suffer from the same food allergy as your family members, you should preferably avoid foods to which they are allergic.

✓ When out shopping, always read food labels to ensure you know what has gone into them. Some products contain gluten; others have nuts in them; still others may contain unknown herbs. If you are allergic to any of them, they could spell trouble for you and your baby.

✓ Unless prescribed by your doctor, avoid taking medication. Drugs, such as oral contraceptives and sedatives, can affect milk production and the baby's sucking reflex.

✓ If the baby shows sensitivity to something in your diet (like refusing to breastfeed or loose stool), consider avoiding it for a few days and see whether that makes a difference. Fish (some kinds contain high levels of mercury), wheat, eggs and nuts are common culprits and may put your baby off breastfeeding.

Plan a Healthy Diet

Stick to a routine

Routine may be boring but sometimes it is necessary. Adopting regular eating habits with specific time intervals ensures that your body gets its quota of energy throughout the day. A good rule of thumb is to have three balanced meals and three snacks.

Make food fun

Healthy meals need not be dull and unimaginative. Go for a varied platter; ensure there is enough texture and colour in your menu and learn the nuances of garnishing your preparations so that they appeal to your senses. Think freshly-chopped coriander leaves sprinkled on dry-cooked vegetables, or tomato and carrot carvings over a rice dish.

Nibble on healthy snacks

How about making space for healthy snacks in your kitchen? That way, when you are hungry, you know you will be reaching out for the right foods. If you think snacks can't be healthy, think fruits, milk, wholegrain crackers, non-buttered popcorn, steamed sprouts, kurmura and khakhras. In cooked options, you have idlis, poha, upma and dalia. Even peanut butter sandwiches will hit the spot when you are yearning for a nibble. Hungry already, aren't you?

Shop and stock wisely

How well you stick to a healthy diet will depend on what you stock up your kitchen with. Cakes and cookies are hardly likely to keep you on track. Nor will ice creams in your fridge. Before you go shopping, draw up a list of things you really need and buy only those: wholegrains, dals, fresh fruits, vegetables, dairy products. Some of these, such as fresh fruits and vegetables, can be stocked on a weekly basis; others, such as milk and milk products, can be replenished daily. Non-vegetarians would do well to freeze their meats in smaller packs for ease of defrosting.

Essential Elements in Your Diet:

Proteins

Proteins are your body's building blocks; they help repair and regenerate muscle tissue. They also benefit the immune system, the bones, organs, and blood. A lack of protein in your diet can impact the quantity of breast milk which you produce. Dangerously low levels can also cause a drop in casein in breast milk. Common sources of proteins are pulses, dairy products, quinoa, fish, chicken, sprouts and seeds, such as sesame and flax.

Consider this: Studies recommend that you consume an additional 25 gm of protein daily in the first six months after delivery and 18 gm during the next six months.

Cereals

They are packed with carbohydrates and provide a boost in energy. But, just as there are good fats and bad fats, there are good carbohydrates and bad carbohydrates. In the former category fall wholegrains with natural fibre—red rice, bajra, ragi, dalia and oats. Bad carbohydrates include maida, polished white rice and other refined grains. In the process of refining they lose their vital nutrients and hence have fewer benefits to offer.

Consider this: Studies recommend about 160–210 gm of carbohydrate intake per day for lactating mothers.

Fruits and vegetables

They provide the bulk of vitamins and minerals in your diet. It is best to have the vegetables raw or lightly cooked since overcooking destroys most of the nutrient content. And have them in a rainbow palette. The colours aren't just great to see, they pack a punch too!

Pinks and reds: Tomatoes, beets, red peppers, watermelon, and grapefruit contain the antioxidant lycopene which is good for your heart, vision, immunity and cells. It also reduces risk of cancer.

Oranges and yellows: Carrots, apricots, peaches, yellow peppers, and squash contain vision-friendly carotenoids.

Greens: Coriander leaves, mint, asparagus, spinach, broccoli, and lettuce contain chlorophyll, a green plant pigment. This pigment is a great source of vitamins, minerals and phytochemicals. So adding greens to the diet fortifies the body against health disorders.

Blues: Grapes, dark berries such as blackberry (*jamun*) and blueberry (*nilabadari*), are packed with the antioxidant anthocyanin which effectively destroys free radicals.

Indigos: Dark berries such as blackberry (*jamun*) and blueberry (*nilabadari*) contain antioxidant bioflavonoids which are antimicrobial, anti-inflammatory, antihistamine and can fight allergies and cancer.

Violets and purples: Beets, brinjals contain betacyanin which improves your immunity.

Fats

If it weren't for small portions of fat in your diet, you probably couldn't withstand the cold. In its absence, your body would find it difficult to absorb vitamins A, D, E and K. Even your hormonal levels would go for a toss if you didn't consume it in adequate quantities. Despite this, fats receive bad publicity and that's mainly because most of us tend to go overboard with our intake, and this leads to obesity and heart problems. Consumed in the right quantities, fats can build cells, provide energy and insulate our organs and nervous system tissue, and that's in addition to all the benefits mentioned above.

No discussion of fats would be complete without the much-publicized good fats and bad fats. And with good reason too! By avoiding bad cholesterol-inducing saturated and trans fats, you will be doing your heart a big favour. Monounsaturated fats, such as olive, peanut and canola oil, as well as polyunsaturated fats, such as corn and sunflower oil, are much healthier as they protect your heart by boosting good cholesterol and sweeping away bad cholesterol. Omega-3 and Omega-6 fatty acids are extremely valuable in brain development; you can get them from fish, walnuts, flaxseeds, and oils such as soya bean and safflower.

Calcium

When you were pregnant you needed extra calcium to help build the bones of the foetus. After delivery, you require it for the production of breast milk. Milk, yoghurt, orange juice, almonds, cheese, sardines, oysters, green vegetables, beans and broccoli are great sources of calcium. If it is possible, supplement your dietary intake with weight-bearing exercises, such as walking or jogging to maintain bone strength.

> **Consider this**: Studies recommend 1,600 mg calcium per day for new mothers.

Vitamin D

Whether or not you assimilate calcium properly also depends on whether or not you have adequate reserves of vitamin D. If you do, your breast milk too will have enough to pass on to the baby. Apart from basking in the early morning rays, you can add to your quota by consuming foods such as milk, egg yolks, tuna and salmon.

> **Consider this**: Lactating mothers need about 5 mcg of vitamin D per day.

Iron

Lactating mothers require the same amount of iron as adult women. Look out for signs such as tiredness and low energy; they may indicate low levels of haemoglobin brought about by an iron deficiency. You can rely on green, leafy vegetables, beans and meats to provide the iron in your diet.

> **Consider this**: You need about 30 mg iron per day.

Water

It is equally important, seeing that the adult body is about 60 to 75 per cent water. A lack of water can cause severe dehydration, headaches, chronic fatigue and even constipation. Not drinking enough water can also impact the production of milk in your breasts.

> **Consider this**: You need to drink about two to three litres of water every day.

	Glossary of Vitamins and Minerals		
Vitamins/ Minerals	*What it does*	*Best food sources*	*Signs of deficiency*
Vitamin A	Antioxidant; promotes healthy eyes and skin, protects against infections and cancer.	Carrots, cabbage, pumpkin, sweet potato, broccoli, liver, eggs, melon, apricots, papaya, spinach, milk.	Poor night vision, dry, flaky skin, frequent colds, acne.
Vitamin C	Strengthens the immune system, absorbs iron, heals wounds, fights infections.	Citrus fruits, tomatoes, strawberries, cabbage, broccoli, melon.	Frequent colds and infection, easy bruising, nose bleeds, tender gums.
Vitamin B12	Helps in formation of red blood cells.	Oysters, tuna, eggs, cottage cheese, cheese, milk, chicken.	Lack of energy, constipation, tender muscles, pale skin, irritability.
Vitamin D	Essential for bone growth and calcium absorption.	Dairy products, fish, egg yolks, sunlight.	Tooth decay, weak bones, hair loss.
Vitamin K	Helps to clot the blood.	Leafy green vegetables, cauliflower, fruits.	
Vitamin E	Needed for blood functioning and fighting free radicals.	Vegetable oils and eggs.	

Vitamins/ Minerals	What it does	Best food sources	Signs of deficiency
Folic Acid	Helps the body use proteins, promotes formation of red blood cells.	Nuts, wholegrains, leafy green vegetables, citrus fruits.	Anaemia, anxiety, lack of energy, poor appetite.
Calcium	Promotes a healthy heart, healthy nerves; improves skin, bones and teeth.	Cheese, almonds, prunes, cooked dried beans, cabbage, pumpkin seeds, dairy products.	Muscle cramps, tooth decay, nervousness.
Potassium	Maintains fluid balance in the body, stimulates gut movements, helps secretion of insulin.	Radish, pumpkin, cauliflower, cabbage, potatoes with skin, bananas, dried fruits, pulses, leafy vegetables.	Nausea, diarrhoea, muscle weakness, irritability.
Magnesium	Strengthens bones and teeth, promotes healthy muscles.	Wheatgerm, almonds, cashew nuts, peanuts, garlic, raisins, green peas, potato skins.	Muscle weakness, lack of appetite, nervousness.
Iron	Forms haemoglobin, vital for producing red blood cells.	Green leafy vegetables, pulses, wholegrains, dried fruits, egg yolks, salmon.	Anaemia, pale skin, fatigue, loss of appetite.
Zinc	Promotes cell growth, bone and tooth formation; heals wounds.	Peanuts, pulses, egg yolks, wholewheat.	Greasy skin, acne, loss of appetite, frequent infections.

To put it in a nutshell

Formulating a healthy diet isn't rocket science. All it needs is common sense and some friendly advice. So here it is, from me to you:

⇒ Eat at regular times every day.
⇒ Start your day with a power-packed breakfast.
⇒ Load up on fruits and vegetables.
⇒ Avoid junk food.
⇒ Ensure variety in food.
⇒ Drink two to three litres of water every day.

5

Exercise and Breastfeeding

Dear Diary,

Today I did what I should have done earlier—stood on the weighing machine and weighed myself. I was horrified by the number that stared back at me. I had heard fancy stories of celebrity new moms who insisted they went back to looking the way they always did simply by exclusive breastfeeding and running about with their babies. Well, dancing to Mia's tunes has done nothing of the sort for me. I am faced with the grim truth—I have got to control my diet and I have got to get into some kind of an exercise regimen. But is it okay for breastfeeding mothers to exercise?

Desperately seeking answers,
S.

To do or not to do—that's the million-dollar question when it comes to exercise, especially when you are still breastfeeding. Of course, as I have already mentioned in Section One, it is advisable to wait until your body recovers completely from the trauma of delivery before you consider putting on your sweats (about four to six weeks). And even after that, it is essential that you take it slow and steady. Going by Srishti's diary entry, it is clear that she had many doubts about the effects of exercise on breastfeeding, which I am sure you have too.

As a new mother, you will have to trust your instincts about how much exercise you can do. That is simple enough, don't you think? Some of you may be too tired from the lack of sleep to enjoy a workout session. In this case, the exercise may actually add to your stress. If so, don't force yourself into it. There will be enough time later to get started. If you do feel up to it, put on your shoes and give in to the delights of this endorphin-releasing activity. If you keep it reasonable, there is no reason why it should interfere with your baby's needs. Just one word of advice: only a breastfeeding mother will truly appreciate the benefits of the correct bra. Choose one that isn't all-elastic, is made of cotton, is roomy enough and provides adequate support.

Many studies that have been conducted in this area show that exercise makes little or no difference to the quality and quantity of breast milk. If you aren't stressed out or tired and if you feel up to it, there's no reason why you shouldn't exercise. In fact, a moderate exercise regimen may make you feel better, less stressed and more in charge of your body. Having said all that, exercise does make additional demands on your body and you must take adequate precautions to ensure that it does not interfere with your or your baby's nutrition. Aim at losing not more than a pound per week.

What you need to know:

✓   Intense exercise can produce a concentration of lactic acid in breast milk, thus giving it a sour taste that can put your baby off drinking.
✓   As it is, breastfeeding your baby means that your body

requires an additional 500-odd calories from your diet. If you exercise, you need to add to those calories to keep up your strength.

✓   Dehydration can affect the amount of milk produced in the breast. Breastfeeding mothers are generally advised to stay well-hydrated and this is even more essential if they are exercising.

How to deal with it:

✓   Feed your infant before exercise. This will prevent the baby's appetite getting spoiled by any lactic acid build-up. Or, give the acid an hour or so after exercise to clear out before nursing.

Cue: The baby suckles happily and for an adequate time.

✓   Don't skimp on calories if you are keen on exercising. Just make sure you are getting them from healthy sources (look in the chapter, *Nutrition and Breastfeeding*).

Cue: The baby puts on adequate weight.

✓   Keep an eye on your urine. If it is pale, you are doing all right. If it turns darker, it means you need to increase your intake of drinking water.
    (*Note:* certain medications can cause the urine to turn dark.)

Cue: The baby is happy after feeding and pees at least five to six times a day.

6
FAQ

Dear Diary,

Life seems to have become one big question mark for me. Every step of the way I am faced with doubts. Should I do this? Or, that? Is this better for my kid? Am I going about it all wrong? It just makes you realize how little one really knows. If only someone would come up with all the answers, it would be a big, big help.

S.

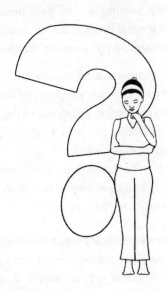

Here are some common queries that new mothers tend to direct at me:

1. ***How often should I feed my baby?***
   It is best to leave that to the baby. The number may be as high as eight to fifteen times a day for the first day or two. This will taper out to six to eight times by the end of week one.

2. ***How will I know whether my baby is getting enough milk?***
   These are the good signs:
   - The baby is feeding six to eight times a day and consequently should go through at least six to eight nappies in that time.
   - His urine should be pale and odourless.
   - His stool should be yellowish.
   - His skin should feel firm. He should make gulping sounds while nursing, get off your breast comfortably after he's done and he should seem content.
   - Your breasts should feel emptier after feeding.

   These are signs that your baby is not getting enough milk:
   - He doesn't gain as much weight as he should.
   - He pees less than six to eight times a day.
   - He passes dark stool just once a day.
   - His skin looks yellow, wrinkled.
   - He demands to be fed constantly, makes clicking sounds while feeding and continues to be cranky afterwards.
   - He seems sleepy all the time.

3. ***Does a vegetarian diet cause protein deficiency?***
   Pure vegetarians need not worry: they can get their daily quota from pulses and grains, milk and milk products,

and soya. Dairy products derived from animal sources are complete proteins. Vegetable proteins need to be combined with other foods to be complete, so one must consume grains with lentils (roti and dal), nuts and seeds and so on.

> Vegetarian items, each of which yields about 7 gm of protein (as much as is contained in 30 gm of meat):
> ¼ cup cottage cheese
> 240 ml milk (8 gm protein)
> ½ cup cooked legumes or lentils
> ½ cup yoghurt
> ¼ cup tofu
> 1 cup soy milk
> 2 tbsp mixed nuts

4. *Is it okay for breastfeeding mothers to drink alcohol, such as wine, beer, hard drinks?*

Alcohol has a way of turning up in breast milk and from there, making its way into your baby's tummy. Even in small quantities this may be dangerous since babies can't metabolize alcohol half as effectively as adults. Studies show that breastfeeding babies whose mothers drink alcohol show a drop in appetite and also appear drowsy (they fall asleep quickly but only for shorter periods of time). Alcohol may also affect their digestion. So, most experts advise mothers to abstain completely during the entire time that they are breastfeeding (or at least for the first three months). But if you must have an occasional drink, here's what you can do:

☞ Restrict yourself to one unit, not more than once or twice a week (1 unit = half a pint of beer, 25 ml of spirit or 125 ml of wine). The more you drink, the longer it will take to clear from your bloodstream. Too much alcohol can also affect the release of breast milk.

☞ Have a bite to eat before you drink and have a glass of water afterwards to ward off dehydration. This helps bring down the amount of alcohol in your blood.

☞ On an average, one unit of alcohol takes about two hours to clear from the bloodstream. So try and nurse your baby immediately before drinking and then a couple of hours afterwards.

5. *I've heard that breastfeeding is the best way to regain one's figure. Is that true?*

Here's an interesting fact which I am sure you didn't know: Breastfeeding burns calories. During the first six months of lactation, a mother produces about 550–1,200 ml milk per day. Since producing 100 ml milk expends about 85 kcal, a healthy, breastfeeding mother can hope to burn calories even while feeding. That's not all. To produce milk, the mother's body utilizes the fat that had been accumulated during pregnancy, making it a great fat-buster. Moreover, as the baby suckles, the mother's system generates hormones which help contract her enlarged uterus and bring the abdomen back into shape faster than in the case of non-breastfeeding mothers. An additional bonus, of course, is that breastfeeding imbues the mother with a sense of calm.

6. *Are there foods that stimulate milk production?*

Yes, they are called lactagogues, and include milk, garlic, almonds and garden cress seeds. Special foods, such as saunth and gond laddoos, are given during lactation.

7. *Is it wise to follow a low-calorie diet during lactation?*

An energy intake of at least 1,800 kcal/day, consisting of nutrient-rich foods, is advisable for lactating women. Lean women are in danger of decreased milk production if they restrict their diet to less than that. Obese women could exclude high-calorie foods but they shouldn't try to lose more than half to one kilogram per week, and that, too, if advised by the doctor. Once the baby is weaned, the mother will no longer need the additional calories and she can safely reduce her food intake and supplement it with an exercise regimen to get back into shape.

Take it from me: Get all the advice you can, but at the same time trust your instincts to guide you during this delicate phase. If you listen hard, your body will tell you just what to eat and how much to exercise. Do that and there's not much chance of your going wrong.

DIET

Weight loss does not happen overnight. If it took nine months of pregnancy for you to deliver a perfectly healthy baby, you must allow a reasonably long (if not longer) time frame to get back into shape. Through this process, your best friends are a healthy diet and regular exercise. In this section, I intend to run you through the fundamental principles of a good diet. Sure, it isn't always easy to watch what you eat—not when there are other, more pressing, issues facing you, and certainly not when you weigh it against the underlying emotional and psychological changes at work during this period. Still, it is something worth aiming for, if only to give you a sense of having some control over your body, and the satisfaction of doing something towards regaining your pre-pregnancy figure. Remember, when the going gets tough, the tough get going.

Note: Before immersing yourself in the following chapters, a word of advice. Any weight loss or diet plan should be undertaken *after* the breastfeeding phase comes to an end. This is because, during breastfeeding, an additional intake of 550 calories is required in the first six months and 400 calories in the subsequent six months after delivery. So don't attempt to cut down on too many calories at the outset. During breastfeeding, the goal should be to eat a healthy, nutritious diet that provides ample nourishment to the baby.

7

Setting Goals

Dear Diary,

I love following the lives of celebrities and have always wondered how they manage to look fit and fabulous at all times. Especially the celebrity mothers who seem to bounce back to their pre-pregnancy shape within a couple of months without breaking into a sweat. I thought I could be like them, except that reality isn't as rosy as the glossies I am used to reading. Nearly four months have passed since delivery and I am no closer to my weight loss goals. I wish I had a magical wand that would zap me back into shape in no time.

S.

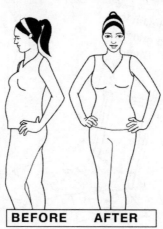

BEFORE   AFTER

Celebrities certainly seem to lead the good life. But what isn't immediately apparent from the glossy pictures in magazines is the amount of effort (at times over the top and unrealistic) which they have to put in just so they can be their slim, slender selves once more, without any evident downtime. For all my clients who wish to emulate these celebrities, I have only one piece of advice: Set realistic weight loss goals—say about a pound (half a kilo) per week, through a combination of diet and exercise. And accept that it might take six months or even longer to return to your pre-pregnancy shape, whether you are breastfeeding or not (weaning your baby early doesn't seem to accelerate weight loss). Even then, your weight might settle down a bit differently from your pre-pregnancy time. Once you accept that and, instead, concentrate on developing a healthy lifestyle, you will be able to take pride in the changes that you see in your body.

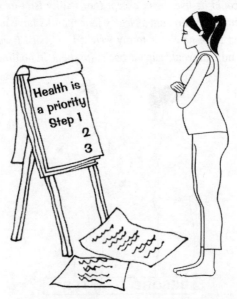

What you need to know:

✓   Why is it such a struggle for a new mother to lose weight? Because nature intended it to be that way. Women's bodies tend to store fat to nourish babies during pregnancy and while breastfeeding. In fact, during the last trimester of pregnancy, new fat cells are added for just this purpose. These cells linger on even after pregnancy, and the most you can hope for is to shrink them with the correct diet and exercise.

✓   During pregnancy you may have gained about 11–14kg (this includes the baby's weight, placenta, amniotic fluid, weight of the enlarged uterus, breast tissue, body fluids and fat stores). Each of these is vital for the baby and the mother.

✓   After delivery, you will find yourself lighter by about 4–5kg. This includes the weight of the baby, placenta and amniotic fluid. There will be more weight loss in the following week as you begin to shed retained fluids. But the one thing that does not disappear like magic are the fat deposits. That will need some work on your part.

How to deal with it:

✓   As far as calorie requirements go, remember that as a breastfeeding mother, you need an additional 550 calories in the first six months and 400 calories in the six months following delivery. So don't attempt to cut down on too many calories at the outset.

✓   Instead of starting off on some fad diet, stick to a healthy eating pattern—low-fat and packed with the recommended vitamins and minerals.

✓   Drink at least eight to ten glasses of water a day.

✓   Be aware of what you eat in order to avoid, and to keep track of, excessive bingeing.

✓   Know the reason for your binges. Are you stressed out? Are you on an emotional roller-coaster? Do you constantly feel low on energy on account of lack of sleep and running around with the baby? If you know the cause of overeating, you can address the issue itself instead of creating a new one—weight gain.

✓   Once in a while, allow yourself a treat without feeling guilty about it.

✓   Stick to a plan which you can follow for the longterm. Crash diets will help in the short run but cannot be sustained for long.

Top Tip for Diet Management

Keep a diary. It is my favourite bit of advice for all who wish to lose weight (which I passed on to Srishti as well). It is a good way to keep track of what and how much you are eating, and it reveals where all those extra calories are coming from—the sugary biscuits at tea; the midnight snack raid; the oily samosas eaten when watching television... A conscientiously maintained diary can hold up a mirror to your eating habits and reveal problems, such as mindless eating, which can make your best weight loss efforts come to naught.

8
Eating Right

Dear Diary,

My friend Sagarika is a fanatic about dieting. Put a plate in front of her and she will start weighing everything on it in terms of calories. 'I have to watch what I eat, after all,' is her common refrain. And she has lost a lot of weight. But do you know something? It doesn't suit her. She looks kind of haggard. Tired, you know. She had such pretty hair and skin, but now it all looks listless. If that's how one looks after dieting, I'd much rather stay away from it.

S.

This is a common mistake most dieters make—they get so involved with the number of calories that they tend to forget their quality. Take it from me, it isn't enough to know *how many* calories you should eat in a day; you should know *what* makes up those calories. And this is where my concept of a balanced meal comes in.

What you need to know:

My concept of a balanced meal is one which includes four important food groups, which are:

- ✓ **Cereals:** They form the bulk of your requirement and contain carbohydrates. They are a major source of energy.
- ✓ **Protein-rich foods:** They help build, repair and maintain muscles, bones, organs, the blood and the immune system.
- ✓ **Fruits and vegetables:** They fulfil different vitamin and mineral requirements.
- ✓ **Fats and sugars:** Sugars provide energy while fats not only provide energy, but preserve body heat and protect the internal organs from damage. They keep your hair and skin healthy; they also help dissolve and absorb vitamins A, D, E and K. Some essential fatty acids are also required to manufacture certain hormones. They are vital but should be taken sparingly.

How to deal with it:

8. Base your three main meals on this concept. On your plate, this will constitute:
    - ☞ **Cereals**—unrefined wholegrains like rice, wheat, barley, bajra, millet, jowar and oats, as well as grain variants, such as poha, sooji and dalia.
    - ☞ **Protein-rich foods**—(vegetarian) low-fat milk and milk products, pulses, dals, sprouts, nuts, seeds, quinoa and soya products; (non-vegetarian) lean meats, especially chicken, fish and egg whites.
    - ☞ **Fruits and vegetables**—a varied colour palette that includes red tomatoes, white cabbage, purple brinjals, yellow peppers, green spinach, orange papaya, green grapes, red watermelon and so on.
    - ☞ **Fats and sugars**—small portions (not more than two spoons a day) of oil and some sugar, preferably natural sugar derived from fruits. Taken in the right quantities,

these will allow you to lose weight without looking haggard.

9.   Skip any one of these and you are missing an important food group. Srishti disliked vegetables and preferred to eat her rotis with dal but by doing so, she was missing out on important vitamins and minerals. So try and incorporate all the elements for that ideal, balanced meal.

Calorie watch

Srishti came up with a good one the other day. 'If I can eat only a certain number of calories a day, what's to stop me from gorging on ice-cream at lunch and then starving for the rest of the day? I am still sticking to the required calorie intake, aren't I?' 'Yes, you are,' I said, 'but what you are doing is satisfying your taste buds, not your body. Ice cream cannot give your body the required nutrients and so is not recommended as a stand-alone meal.' She thought she had spotted a loophole in my reasoning but, as I explained to her—much to her disappointment—mere calorie control isn't enough; it is important to ensure that those calories are culled from the four major food groups that represent my concept of a balanced meal. 'There goes my ice cream meal,' she pouted.

So, exactly how many calories are there in a roti? Is naan better or paratha? For all those who are stuck with the math, here is an easy calorie chart based on the balanced meal. Srishti has stuck it on her fridge door and uses it to plan healthy, low-calorie menus for her family.

Note:
Minimum calorie intake a day for a breastfeeding mother: 1,800
Minimum calorie intake a day for a mother who is not breastfeeding: 1,200
This minimum calorie requirement will increase if you are leading an active life and exercising regularly.

Cereals

2 slices of bread	150 calories
1 roti	70 calories
1 paratha	235 calories
1 naan	150 calories
2 khakhras	120 calories
1 cup rice (40 gm)	140 calories
1 cup oat porridge	150 calories
1 cup cereal flakes	185 calories
1 serving of noodles (75 gm)	240 calories
1 serving of wholewheat pasta (75 gm)	200 calories

Protein-rich Foods

Dairy and Egg

1 cup cow's milk (200 ml)	135 calories
1 cup buffalo's milk (200 ml)	230 calories
1 cup skimmed milk (200 ml)	60 calories
1 cup buttermilk (200 ml)	50 calories
1 cup low-fat yoghurt (150 ml)	60 calories
100 gm cottage cheese (paneer)	250 calories
1 medium-sized egg	80 calories
3 egg whites	50 calories

Nuts

10 almonds (10 gm)	100 calories
7 cashew nuts (20 gm)	120 calories
20 peanuts (10 gm)	60 calories
10 pistachios (10 gm)	65 calories

Pulses (Dals)

1 cup plain dal	150 calories
1 cup chick peas (channa)	250 calories

Meat and Fish (cooked with minimal oil)

1 cup mutton curry	295 calories
2 pieces tandoori chicken	175 calories
1 cup fish curry	250 calories

1 cup prawn curry	327 calories
1 medium piece chicken breast/fish	100 calories
1 bowl chicken soup	110 calories

Fruits/Vegetables

Fruits

1 large apple (100 gm)	60 calories
1 small banana (200 gm)	100 calories
1 small mango (100 gm)	74 calories
20 grapes (100 gm)	71 calories
1 slice melon (100 gm)	20 calories
1 medium orange (100 gm)	72 calories
1 medium peach (100 gm)	50 calories
1 medium pear (150 gm)	75 calories
1 slice papaya (100 gm)	30 calories
1 slice pineapple (100 gm)	50 calories
1 cup pomegranate (100 gm)	70 calories

Vegetables (Salad)

1 medium carrot (60 gm)	29 calories
1 medium capsicum (100 gm)	24 calories
1 medium cucumber (150 gm)	20 calories
100 gm lettuce	20 calories
1 medium onion (50 gm)	25 calories
1 medium tomato (60 gm)	10 calories
1 small radish (150 gm)	25 calories

Cooked Vegetables (with minimal oil)

1 cup green vegetables	90 calories
1 cup mixed vegetables	120 calories
1 cup brinjal	185 calories
1 cup potato (dumaloo)	200 calories

Vegetable Soups

1 bowl tomato soup	60 calories
1 bowl mushroom soup	110 calories
1 bowl minestrone soup (with noodles)	130 calories

Fats and Sugars

Oils

1 tsp butter (5 gm)	36 calories
1 tsp ghee (5 gm)	45 calories
1 tsp oil (5 gm)	40 calories

Sugar

1 tsp white sugar (5 gm)	20 calories
1 tsp honey (5 gm)	15 calories
Jaggery (5 gm)	19 calories

Accompaniments

1 tsp jam	30 calories
1 tsp pickle	35 calories
1 tbsp tomato ketchup	17 calories
1 tbsp mayonnaise	150 calories
1 tbsp French dressing	70 calories

Top Tips for Balanced Meals

⇒ Opt for unrefined grains. In the process of refining, most grains lose their fibre and valuable nutrients.

⇒ It is a good idea to include soya in your diet. Despite being derived from a plant, it contains all nine essential amino acids in sufficient proportions to be considered a complete protein.

⇒ When it comes to eggs, it is best to stick to egg whites since the yolk is high in fat and cholesterol.

⇒ Avoid overcooking vegetables if you want to retain their nutrients. Have them lightly stir-fried instead.

⇒ Be wary of packaged goods because they are often packed with preservatives and too much sugar or salt.

9
Eat Little, Eat Often

Dear Diary,

I thought the whole point of going on a diet was to STOP eating. So when Namita told me to have three balanced meals and 3–4 snacks in between, I stopped and stared. Had I heard her right? Was she joking? As it turns out, the joke's on me. The best way to lose weight, she explained, is to eat little but often. It will keep my energy levels up and, at the same time, boost my metabolism enough to spur weight loss. I am sure there's a catch somewhere that defines what exactly it is that one can eat, but at least it means no starvation. I don't think I would have handled that well at all.

S.

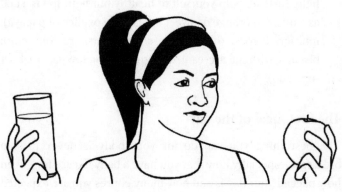

As I told Srishti, sticking to three large meals a day doesn't help your diet anyway. Instead, it makes sense to emulate the French and eat little, eat often, through the course of the day.

What you need to know:

✓ Large meals are unnecessary. They are harder to digest and make you feel sluggish and low on energy.

✓ The longer periods of starving that follow these large meals cause a drop in blood sugar levels and induce food cravings which can upset the diet applecart.

✓ Smaller meals eaten through the day are a much better bet. They keep your body's metabolism burning, thereby boosting weight loss.

How to deal with it:

✓ Aside from three balanced meals (had in moderation), eat three to five snacks a day, once every two to three hours.

✓ Apart from the frequency, the emphasis here is on having bite-sized portions, not mouthfuls. *What* you are eating also matters. Gorging on samosas and kachoris isn't going to help. Instead, help yourself to healthy but light foods, such as fruits, (an orange or sweet lime, apple or slice of papaya); multigrain toast (one to two slices); kurmura (one cup); biscuits without a cream filling (two); or low-fat yoghurt (one cup).

The first meal of the day

The best thing you can do for your body is never to skip breakfast, especially now that you have a baby to care for. Given how packed your day is and how many chores you are expected to perform, a hearty breakfast is just the thing you need. It fuels your body after a night-long period of fasting and helps kick-start your day. So make it the first of several mini meals you will have throughout the day. And, what exactly constitutes a healthy breakfast? Foods high in fibre: fresh whole fruits; multigrain cereals, such as oats, wheat, ragi and jowar; lightly steamed vegetables and sprouts, skimmed milk and low-fat dairy products. You don't need to come up with complex recipes—a slice of wholewheat bread with low-fat cottage cheese and sliced tomatoes and cucumbers is a healthy dish. So is cereal with low-fat milk and fresh fruits. Hot dishes, such as poha and upma aren't time-consuming if you do a little bit of advance preparation, such as roasting the rawa the previous night.

When the craving hits

Small, frequent meals should put the stopper on your cravings but if you do get one, it is all right to give in occasionally. Rate the craving on a scale of 1–10 where 10 represents the most urgent craving and, if it looks like it's veering towards the two-digit number, satisfy it. But do so sensibly. Sit down at the dining table. Take a small portion of whatever it is you are craving for, say, a slice of chocolate cake. Slowly savour every tiny bite. That way, you feel satisfied with much less. Never binge on the move or stand in front of the refrigerator for you will only end up overeating. If your craving falls much lower on the scale, try distraction techniques. Call up a friend for a good chat. Brush your teeth. Drink water. Watch a movie. If it is stress that is making you feel hungry, resolve the issue instead of reaching out for that packet of chips. Do this and you will realize that your craving has passed.

Healthy snack substitutes

✓ Instead of ice cream try sherbet, ice golas or low-fat fruit yoghurt.

✓ Longing for chocolate? Try chocolate-flavoured skimmed milk.

✓ If you are craving for something sweet, try a digestive biscuit topped with jam.

✓ Replace farsans and fried snacks with kurmura and non-buttered popcorn.

✓ Avoid aerated drinks. Stick to herbal teas, lime juice, coconut water or plain water.

✓ Sprinkle chaat masala on fruits and salads to make them interesting.

Top Tips to Snacking Right

⇒ Have ready-to-eat, healthy options at hand for snacking.

⇒ Eat at fixed times, and that includes snacks.

⇒ Focus on the food which you are eating.

⇒ Never eat on the move.

⇒ If you *must* have packaged foods, make wise choices after reading the labels. Keep a lookout for dangers like transfats, saturated fats and high cholesterol.

10

Water Matters

Dear Diary,

I have never been much of a water drinker. I can manage 2–3 glasses a day at the most. It is not like I am depriving my body, I just don't feel thirsty and if my body did need water, it would tell me, right? But Namita believes it is time to change things. I need to drink more to ensure adequate breast milk production. That aside, more water in my system will prevent toxins from building up in my body, make my hair and skin glow, and help me lose weight. H'm, all great reasons to give it a try. So, two litres of water it is for me, starting tomorrow.

S.

Most people to whom I talk are worried about the food they eat—what kind, how much, how often. But few, if any, give thought to water. That is surprising, considering that it is an essential part of a good diet and that it can actually help you towards attaining your weight loss goals. Drinking water is especially important for new mothers. It provides hydration at a time when their bodies are utilizing all available resources to produce milk for the baby. So drink up, new mothers!

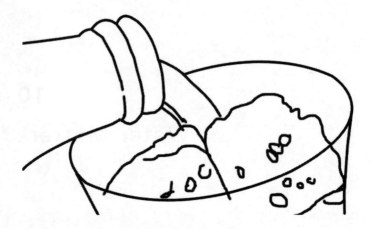

What you need to know:

✓ It is sad but true, most people drink only about three to four glasses of water a day—that's half of what they actually require. This is strangely at variance with the fact that our body constitutes 65–70 per cent water.

✓ Drinking water has many benefits: It keeps your kidneys functioning effectively, prevents toxin build-up and adds a glow to your skin, eyes and hair. It aids weight loss too by suppressing your appetite. Sometimes, what you think is a food craving is just your body asking for water; so, drink up and you will feel the craving pass.

✓ Dehydration, especially in new mothers, can cause low blood pressure, constipation, poor metabolism and decreased milk production. Since it hampers digestion and proper bowel movement, it also makes it more difficult for them to knock off those extra pounds.

✓ New mothers who are embarking on an exercise regimen to get back into shape need even more water to make up for the loss of water through perspiration.

✓ A good indicator of whether or not you are drinking enough water is the colour of your urine. If it is pale yellow, almost clear, you are drinking enough. If it is darker, you need to increase your quota (do check with your doctor first since some medications can cause urine to change colour).

How to deal with it:

✓ Start your day with two glasses of water. If you like, have it warm and with lemon juice added to it. This makes a great start to the day.

✓ Thereafter, keep drinking water—preferably a total of about 8–12 glasses or about 2–3 litres—through the day.

✓ If you are averse to drinking so much water, you can include green tea or coconut water.

Top Tips for Drinking Up

⇒ Keep a water bottle handy wherever you are. Sip on it while you are nursing to keep dehydration at bay.

⇒ Even when you are exercising, take breaks every thirty minutes to sip water. It will help replace fluid loss through perspiration.

⇒ Have water with your meals.

⇒ Sip water even when you aren't really thirsty. It is believed that thirst is an indication that your body is already dehydrated.

⇒ To ensure you are drinking enough, fill your quota of bottles every morning (despite all the distractions) and make sure you run through them by the end of the day.

⇒ Eat fresh fruits and vegetables, such as oranges, sweet limes, musk melons, watermelons, tomatoes and cucumbers which are high in water content.

11

Eat Light at Night

Dear Diary,

I spend so much time with Mia these days that come dinner time I am dying for some adult company. But my husband returns from work pretty late, and I like to wait to have dinner with him. These get-togethers are very comforting for me. Talking over a hot dinner about the day's events, in particular of Mia's latest antics, is almost enough to erase all signs of fatigue. And since that's the only time he eats at home, I make sure there is interesting food on the table. Nothing like a full, content stomach to end the day with, right?

S.

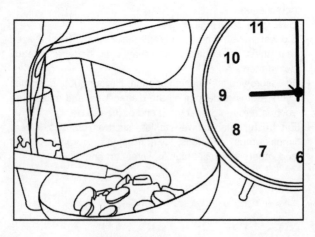

For all those of you who are struggling to lose pregnancy weight, I have only one question to ask: What are you eating after 9 p.m.? Seems like an innocuous question, but in that answer lies the real story behind your weight loss (or lack of it).

What you need to know:

Timing of meals is everything. At the end of a long day your physical activity tapers off. You are tired. Your energy levels are low. And your body is gearing up to retire for the night. What you need is a nice, light meal at this point—just enough to induce sound sleep but not enough to let the food lie in your stomach undigested. Stuff yourself with too many calories at this hour—you may be tempted to, you may even feel you deserve it after a long, tiring day looking after your baby—and you are laying the groundwork for more weight gain.

How to deal with it:

✓ The ideal way is to avoid eating altogether after nine. Why nine, you may ask? Because it gives your digestive system a couple of hours to work before you go to bed. If you tend to sleep earlier, you need to time your last meal of the day accordingly—that is, at least two hours before bedtime.

✓ Sure, some of you may think this deadline impractical, since many families get together only post-nine to have dinner together, as in Srishti's case. In that case, it is best to eat light at this time. Less of fried foods, buttery sauces and creamy gravies. More salads, grilled and roasted dishes. And avoid second helpings. It is easy amid the laughter and chatter of your family to lose track of what exactly you are tucking into, so stay focused. Try and stay awake for at least two hours afterwards.

✓ I remember Srishti asking me, 'But just what is meant by eating light?' It means eating low-fat food and keeping 20 percent of your stomach empty, I told her (refer to Chapter 10 of this section for more information). It keeps you satisfied but not overly stuffed. If you've eaten light, you'll find yourself more than willing to go for a stroll. If not, you'll be hard-pressed even to leave the table. Adhere to this rule and you will notice a considerable difference in your weight.

Top Tips for Eating Light

⇒ Eat slowly.
⇒ Put your fork down after every bite to ensure you chew every morsel.
⇒ Focus all your attention on the food before you. That means no reading or watching television when eating.
⇒ Don't linger after you've finished eating.
⇒ Use smaller plates.
⇒ Avoid keeping serving dishes on the table in front of you for this will only tempt you to go for a second helping.
⇒ Swap lighter foods for heavier foods

12
Eating Out

Dear Diary,

These days I just don't feel like cooking elaborate meals. If I had the choice, I would eat out every day. Ah, the pleasure of having someone serving piping hot food that I haven't had to labour over! It would be a good change of scene for me too, away from all the frantic activity surrounding Mia. The only thing that keeps me from even considering that option is the fear that I will not be able to control myself, I will end up consuming many more calories than is good for me. As if I need more reasons for freaking out!

S.

Cooking takes up a lot of time—planning meals, shopping for groceries, prepping, cooking and serving. And while you manage it with a little help on most days—with one eye firmly on the baby as you potter about the kitchen—it is but natural to feel the occasional need to ditch it all and dine out. Simple, except that you feel guilty about all the calories that you would inevitably tuck into during a night out. But dining out need not be the guilt-ridden experience that you've come to expect it to be, that is, if you indulge only occasionally and if you know how to be smart about your choices.

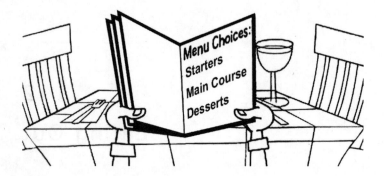

What you need to know:

✓   Restaurant food, such as maida breads and rotis, is usually heavy on oil, cream, butter and refined products, but most establishments are open to special food requests from patrons. Make the most of it.

✓   Learn to read between the lines of the menu so that you can eliminate foods which are dangerous for your waistline. If in doubt, always discuss your choices with the waiter.

How to deal with it:

✓   Look for fibre-rich, wholegrain breads in the bread basket. The fibre present in wholegrain foods is filling and nutritious.

✓   Order nimbupani, coconut water or buttermilk on the side instead of alcohol and aerated drinks.

✓   Fill up on a fibre-rich salad with low-calorie dressing, and a vegetable soup with toasted croutons before moving on to the next course.

✓   Order light foods and smaller helpings for the main course. Stick to steamed, baked and grilled dishes, and ask for rich sauces to be served on the side so that you can monitor how much you are consuming. At all times be aware of what you are tucking into.

✓ Finish your meal with some herbal mint tea: it is good for digestion. If, for dessert, you *must* have a chocolate dish, share it with your family instead of having all of it. Opt for lighter foods when possible, such as sorbets or fresh fruits.

✓ At a buffet, use a smaller plate to keep you from piling food on it.

Eat global

Many international cuisines offer low-calorie options for a gourmet dieter like you. Consider these options:

Indian: tandoori foods, steamed idlis, raitas, kachumbars, lentils, vegetables without cream gravies.

Thai/Chinese: stir-fried vegetables, steamed wontons, steamed fish, clear soups.

Mexican: tostadas, taco salads (preferably without the shell or if with shell, baked instead of fried), beans, vegetables, grilled lean meats, salsa.

Italian: tomato-based sauces, wholewheat pastas/pizzas with lots of vegetables, grilled lean meats.

Japanese: sushi, tofu, yakimono (a Japanese term for dishes which are grilled, pan-fried or broiled), no tempura please.

Lebanese: tabouleh, wheat pita bread, dips such as hummus, muhammara, harissa (say no to deep-fried falafel and kebabs).

Top Tips for Eating Out

⇒ *Do* ask for minimal oil to be used for stir-fry, sauté and tadka cooking techniques. Olive oil may be healthier, but it still contains calories. Use sparingly.

⇒ *Don't* gorge on on-the-house buttery breads.

⇒ *Do* choose fresh lime soda with salt or less sugar syrup.

⇒ *Don't* go for vegetables with fat-laden sauces or gravies and preparations swimming in heavy, full-cream bases, ghee or butter.

⇒ *Do* order dishes with fresh fruits, sprouts, salad vegetables, raita or low-fat paneer.

⇒ *Don't* have oily kulchhas and parathas. Have dry tandoori rotis instead.

⇒ *Do* order tomato-based sauces instead of cheesy sauces.

⇒ *Don't* be tempted by cheesy pizzas. Order them without or with half the cheese. You could also try a tomato-based, cheese-less version.

⇒ *Do* try wholewheat or multigrain bread in sandwiches.

⇒ *Don't* order sandwiches dripping with butter or mayonnaise.

⇒ *Do* include moong dal, moong sprouts or some other lentil if you are vegetarian. It adds to the protein component to your meal.

⇒ *Don't* choose fried rice when you can have steamed rice.

⇒ *Do* opt for grilled/tandoori chicken and fish if you are non-vegetarian.

13

Eat, Don't Overeat

Dear Diary,

For me, food is an indicator of how my day has gone. I am usually able to control my binges if everything is running smoothly and nothing has happened to upset my emotional balance. But God forbid if something should go wrong! I make a beeline for the kitchen to lay my hands on anything that I can get. Tub of ice cream. Packet of chips. If nothing else, gobs of butter. How am I going to stick to my diet if I keep overeating on the slightest pretext? I cannot control circumstances and make sure everything is going to be all right all the time.

Help,
S.

People eat when they are happy. They eat when they are down in the dumps. They eat because they are stressed out. And because they realize they aren't losing weight as fast as they want to. Some people even eat just because the food is there—demanding to be eaten. And because it is too expensive (why waste it?) or too cheap (might as well make the most of it!). By Srishti's own admission, she had used one or the other of these excuses to gorge on food at some point. She thought it made her feel better. In reality, she was only piling on calories and making it harder for her to lose weight.

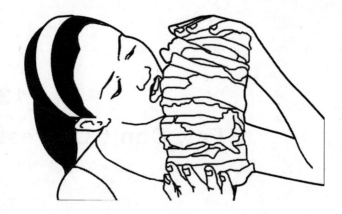

What you need to know:

Eat at regular intervals. The longer the gap between meals, the hungrier you get. This means the more you are likely to overeat. If you stick to just this one basic principle, you will save your system from getting overburdened.

How to deal with it:

- ✓ Don't use your stomach as a dumping ground for leftovers. Store them in the fridge instead.
- ✓ If you think it's a waste to leave food on your plate, make it a habit to take smaller helpings. Forcing yourself to finish something isn't good for your system.
- ✓ Not now, but when your baby grows up, you may feel bound to finish off what's left on his plate. Not a good idea.
- ✓ Avoid super-size meals in fast-food chains. They might seem like good value for money but they certainly aren't good for you.
- ✓ Always be aware of *how much* you are eating—especially if you are hanging out with friends or catching a movie.

✓ No matter how delectable and varied the spread in front of you is, choose what you like most and have just that in moderation. If you must try everything, do so with a spoon, not a plateful.

✓ It is best not to keep tempting foods within easy reach. If you see them, you will have them.

✓ If you *must* indulge, do so while sitting down and have only a small portion. When out with friends, make it a point to share a sinful treat with them rather than have it all by yourself.

✓ Just because something is low-fat and low-cal is no reason to overeat. It *does* pack calories.

✓ Don't use your emotions as a justification for eating. Happy? Go buy a new dress for yourself. Sad? Watch a funny movie. Stressed out? Go for a brisk walk. It isn't healthy to resolve everything with food.

Fast Food, Junk Food

It is difficult to keep away from junk food, but it does no favours to your system. While I wouldn't rule out an occasional indulgence, it would be ideal to consider other options as well:

✓ Give a healthy twist to junk food at home with wholewheat pizzas and pastas with tomatoes and vegetables, and roti rolls with a spicy potato filling instead of frankies.

✓ Avoid fast-food joints and haunt salad bars and juice parlours instead.

✓ Instead of the packaged foods that you usually stock up at home, try healthier alternatives, such as fresh fruits, wholegrain granola bars, crackers and yoghurt.

✓ Try substitution. Instead of a cream biscuit, have a digestive biscuit. Instead of ice cream, have a cup of flavoured yoghurt.

Instead of fried farsan, have roasted khakhras or savouries, such as kurmura, popcorn, and other low-fat baked snacks (check in health stores for innovative low-fat, tasty options). Instead of coffee with full-fat milk, have skimmed milk decaf, green tea or coconut water.

Here's a calorie chart for junk food

1 plate samosas (2 pieces)	320 calories
1 plate paprichaat (6–8 pieces)	260 calories
1 plate alootikki (2 pieces)	320 calories
1 plate assorted pakodas (8 pieces)	360 calories
1 plate instant noodles or pasta (100 grams)	460 calories
1 plate seekh kebabs (2–3 pieces)	260 calories
1 plate paneer tikka (8 pieces)	370 calories
1 plate bread with jam (2 slices)	260 calories
1 plate masala dosa	470 calories
1 plate idli-sambhar	300 calories
1 plate vada-sambhar	400 calories
1 plate pav bhaji	420 calories
1 plate assorted namkeen (fried savouries)	650 calories
1 plate cheesy garlic bread (2 pieces)	510 calories
1 plate chowmein	300 calories
1 small packet wafers	550 calories

Constipation? Drive it out!

If you're eating all right and still feel that your system is overburdened, constipation may be to blame. Most new mothers may face the problem immediately after delivery—mainly due to soreness in the region and due to fear of pain or splitting of stitches—but if your bowel movements continue to be irregular even afterwards, your weight loss goals may get stuck too! To get them going smoothly, here's what you can do:

✓ Make sure your diet is rich in fibre (about 25–30 gm a day). Dietary fibre is found in fruits, vegetables, sprouts and wholegrain cereals. They contain roughage that eases the process of elimination. Major bowel-friendly foods include figs, prunes, raisins, papaya, pineapple, mint and yoghurt.

✓ Drink plenty of water.

✓ Eat slowly, chewing each morsel to ensure proper digestion.

✓ Exercise regularly.

✓ Use laxatives such as Isabgol only as a last resort and on the doctor's advice.

Top Tips to Avoid Excess

⇒ Don't eat as if food were going out of fashion.

⇒ Eat slowly, chew well, stop when you're *nearly* full.

⇒ Learn to say no when it matters.

14

Know When to Stop

Dear Diary,

If nothing else, my diet is going to make a globetrotter out of me. Why, you ask. First, Namita asked me to emulate the French and eat little but often. Now she is recommending that I take lessons from the Japanese. Japanese? To which she replied, 'Hara hachi bu.' Do I have to take language lessons to decode that?

S.

No, no language lessons needed, I promise. I am always looking for new ideas to add greater value to my dietary suggestions and when I heard of this Japanese phrase, I adopted it immediately. Roughly translated, 'Hara hachi bu' contains some sage dietary

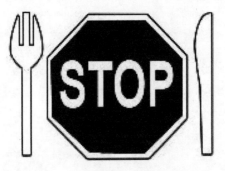

advice: 'Eat until you are 80 per cent full.' It is believed to have come from the very calorie-conscious Okinawans who mouth the phrase before they sit down to their meal. By doing so, they avoid falling into the very trap most weight-watchers find themselves in—not knowing when to stop eating.

What you need to know:

✓ It takes about twenty minutes for your stomach to send signals to your brain that it is full. This time lapse increases the risk of overeating by failing to give you more immediate signals.

✓ If you pay close attention to the food which you are eating instead of just wolfing it down, you can usually prevent stuffing yourself.

How to deal with it:

✓ Take a leaf from the Japanese and go the 80/20 route. Once you get into the habit of leaving your stomach 20 per cent empty, you will not overshoot your stomach's capacity.

✓ Eat slowly, chewing every morsel carefully before swallowing. This allows your system enough time to send out the right signals.

✓ If your plate is empty, don't rush to refill it. Wait a while. Or walk away from the table. Engage yourself in something else. Chances are that you will realize in twenty minutes that you are have had enough and don't need to eat more.

Feel the food

As I keep telling my clients, *how* you eat is as important as *what* you eat. So keep all your baby-linked worries aside during mealtimes and pay attention to your food. Think about its texture, aroma, colour and flavour and take it all in with every bite. It makes for a very satisfying experience—and without the second helping too! Ensure that you eat slowly, in peace and quiet, without the blare of the television to distract you and without getting into emotionally charged chats with the family. Focusing on the task at hand—eating—prevents you from overindulging by letting you know when your stomach is full. It also promotes effective digestion.

Overeating: The Pitfalls

If your trousers feel tight at the waist and you need to lower the zipper in order to ease the pressure, you've probably eaten too much. Many of us equate satiety with being stuffed. In fact, Indian hospitality demands that you feed your guest until he can eat no more—a practice that is responsible for many bulging waistlines! But overeating has its pitfalls and can trigger the following reactions:

- Indigestion
- Gas/ bloating
- Acidity/ heartburn
- Nausea/ vomiting
- Chest discomfort

Top Tips to Stop in Time

⇒ Eat your meals in a peaceful environment. Avoid eating when you are upset.
⇒ Stop eating while there is still some space in your stomach.
⇒ Sit quietly for a few minutes after finishing your meal.
⇒ Stay upright after eating.
⇒ Chew every bite twenty times.

15
The Cleansing Diet Plan

Dear Diary,

To err is human and I seem to be more human than everybody else. How else do you explain the countless times that I have deviated from my diet this last week? On Monday, my parents dropped by and they brought mithai for me. I was eating it all of Tuesday and Wednesday. On Thursday, my husband decided I deserved a break and ordered a pizza with some garlic bread. I gorged on it without restraint. How am I even going to face Namita after this binge? Looks like I am going to end up fat and frumpy.

Several pounds heavier already,
S.

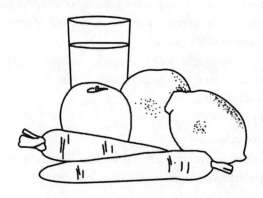

So you went out and binged last night. Try as much as you like, you will not be able to undo that. But you could initiate some damage control to ensure that all is not lost. Here is a one-day SOS cleansing diet plan designed to save your diet.

What you need to know:

✓ This cleansing diet is intended to monitor your food intake so as to give your digestive system a break.

✓ This isn't a daily plan. It is to be followed *once* a week and only *if* you have indulged.

How to deal with it:

Breakfast

✓ Warm herbal tea

✓ Fresh fruits (no mangoes, bananas, custard apples, grapes or chikoos)

Mid-morning

✓ Buttermilk (made with skimmed-milk yoghurt)

Lunch

✓ Vegetable soup or vegetable juice (choose vegetables such as tomatoes, spinach, carrots, celery, bottle gourd, ridge gourd and snake gourd)

✓ Mixed vegetable salad (include tomatoes, cucumbers, lettuce, carrot and celery) with 2 tbsp lightly steamed moong sprouts

Evening

✓ Coconut water

✓ One cup porridge (oatmeal/broken wheat) or a bowl of citrus fruits (oranges, sweet lime, grapefruit)

After-dinner

✓ Herbal tea (chamomile)

✓ One bowl of watermelon

Note: i. Please do not follow this plan if you are breastfeeding.

ii. Drink eight to ten glasses of water along with this diet to aid elimination.

Top Tips to Tackle Bingeing

⇒ Binges happen. Don't get stuck on that, learn to move on.

⇒ Aside from this cheater's cleansing diet, stick to lighter food and a more active exercise schedule for the next couple of days.

⇒ Drink lots of water. It will fill you up and also ensure that your body functions efficiently.

16

Fat Chance!

Dear Diary,

This is exactly one of those things that put a dampener on your spirits! Did you know that a woman's body develops additional fat cells during pregnancy? And that, no matter how hard she tries, she can never be rid of them ever again? It's as if nature is conspiring against us women, to ensure that we have a difficult time losing all that excess fat. Makes me question the wisdom of denying myself food and making an effort to exercise! Why bother when nature itself seems to be working against us?

Grumpily,
S.

The extra fat cells about which Srishti is griping develop towards the end of pregnancy for a reason—to provide nourishment to your baby. While it is a fact that once formed, you cannot change the number of fat cells in your body, you can certainly work on shrinking them in size by reducing your fat intake. And that is never easy, given that it comes in the most

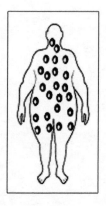

tempting of forms—jalebis, puris, samosas and kachoris. To really understand the effect that fat has on your body, think of it as a car. Just as its fuel tank will overflow if you put in too much petrol, your system will brim over with fat if you consume too much of it. Now, where the car is concerned, the excess petrol simply flows away. But in your body it is stored in your fat cells which will keep expanding to make room for the additional fat. And when they can do that no more, they will simply multiply to keep up.

What you need to know:

✓ One gram of fat equals nine calories. By comparison, one gram of carbohydrates or proteins equals four calories. It goes without saying then that any serious dieter should work on restricting her fat intake to bring down the overall calorie consumption.

✓ Fat fact: one chapati contains ninety calories. A large spoonful of ghee spread over it doubles the calorie count to 180 calories!

✓ Having said all that, a little fat is essential to every diet. So don't eliminate it completely. To be safe, ensure that your fat consumption is about 10 per cent of your daily calorie intake (not more than 2 teaspoons).

✓ Even among fats, there are good fats and bad fats. Unlike the bad fats (mainly saturated fats and transfats) which increase cholesterol, the good monounsaturated and polyunsaturated fats, consumed in limited quantities, are known to reduce blood cholesterol and protect against heart disease.

How to deal with it:

✓ It is easy to avoid visible fats, such as oil, butter, ghee and margarine. But you must look out for the hidden fats as well. They come in several guises—cheese and paneer (they could contain up to 70 per cent milk fat); oily fish, such as tuna and sardines; certain vegetables, such as olives and avocados; processed foods, such as pastries and cookies. Choose your oils with care. Monounsaturated oils, such as olive, peanut and canola, are the best, followed by polyunsaturated oils, such as corn and sunflower.

✓ Learn to think differently when cooking. It isn't the oil that makes a dish delicious; it is the herbs and spices that add flavour to it. So why not limit the use of oil and rely on spices to do the trick?

Top Tips to Go Low-fat

⇒ Dairy products, such as milk, cream, cheese, yoghurt, buttermilk, butter and ghee are high in saturated fats. To derive their benefits without consuming too much, switch to low-fat milk and milk products. To obtain low-fat milk, boil regular milk two to three times. Each time, remove the cream that floats on top so that you end up with low-fat or nearly fat-free milk. Or, use skimmed milk powder and water to obtain low-fat milk. Use this variant to prepare yoghurt, buttermilk and cottage cheese.

⇒ Move away from traditional oils, such as coconut oil, ghee, butter and palm kernel oil. Switch to the much healthier olive, peanut or canola oils. Opt for steaming, grilling or roasting rather than frying when cooking.

⇒ Cultivate the habit of reading labels when out buying groceries. Steer away from products containing transfats, and gravitate towards words like low-fat, non-fat, zero transfat, or 3 gm of fat or less per serving.

17

Mind Your Mind

Dear Diary,

I have to have that piece of cake in the fridge.
No, you don't.
How can I not eat it? It's so gooey and chocolate-y.
You are strong. You can overcome the craving.
How about just a single bite? No one will know.
But you will. And you will feel guilty about it later.
But no one else will have it. No one in the house likes chocolate. It will waste away in the fridge.
Give it away then.
Fine! Have it your way. I will go watch that episode of The Big Bang Theory *instead.*

S.

Sounds familiar? Most dieters encounter moments that will tempt them to yield to their cravings. Whether they overcome them or not will depend on how steadfast their minds are. The greater their

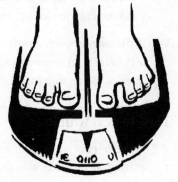

will power, the easier it is to distract them from food. For once, Srishti found herself on the winning side. And for her, who has always found it difficult to control her cravings, this was a sweet victory (pun intended!).

What you need to know:

✓ You may blame it on evolution if you like, but your brain is wired to store body fat in case of drought or famine. Call it saving for a rainy day! As such, resisting food is actually going against nature.

✓ If you intend to lose weight, then you must learn to control your mind. Once your mind decides that you *will* stop overeating, your body will have no choice but to obey.

✓ Here's a small quiz to determine just how strong your mind is. Answer yes or no to the following questions:
    i.   I can never stick to a diet for more than a few days.
    ii. I end up overeating at every meal.
    iii. If there is nothing to do, I eat.
    iv. I eat when I am stressed.
    v.   I can never say no to food, even if I have just eaten.
    vi. I have no time to eat frequently.
    vii. I am too busy to exercise.
    viii. Low-calorie foods are so uninteresting.

✓ If the answers are mostly yes, boy, does your mind need a makeover! If the answers are mostly no, you are on the right track to losing weight.

How to deal with it:

✓ Make a pact with yourself and set down your goals in writing. If possible, also announce them to your friends. A public commitment is more likely to be effective for it holds you accountable to more than just yourself; moreover, you will find it easier to stick to your regimen rather than to lose face in public. Plus, you can always rely on those friends for support when you need them most.

✓ Make a fresh start. If you have had failures before, don't let them deter you from trying again. Instead, learn from them. Identify where you made the mistakes and correct them. Analyse circumstances that caused you to binge in the past so that you know better this time around. The worst thing you can do is give up.

✓ Think of your goal as a reward. Every time you feel tempted to gorge on something fried or sweet, ask yourself if it will help you get your reward. If it won't, would it be worth the momentary satisfaction that you will get from it? Or can you do better and satisfy yourself with a piece of fruit?

✓ Keep telling yourself you can do it. It may sound hollow at first but, as you build on small successes and grow in confidence, it will take on a more convincing ring and lead you to sure-fire victory.

Top Tips to Control Your Mind

⇒ Stay positive. It can give you the most amazing results. It will make you more focused and single-minded in your approach. Always look on the bright side. Never say, 'I've lost only two pounds.' Instead, say, 'I've lost two pounds and I feel great.' This will help keep you on track.

⇒ Keep stress away. Think thin but don't stress about being fat. Stress will only make you reach out for those comfort foods and then, where will you be diet-wise?

18

Don't Be a Yo-Yo

Dear Diary,

Ritu, my sister, is getting married and I am so happy for her. I am excited at the prospect of shopping—new clothes, lots of jewellery, shoes, bags, the works! I am so tempted to do something drastic to lose all that extra weight around my tummy—like, starve myself to get into shape, just for the duration of the wedding, you know? But is that healthy?

S.

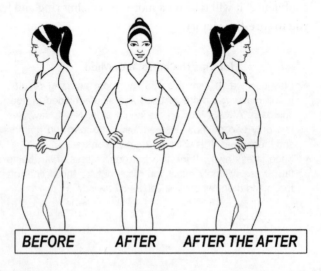

BEFORE   AFTER   AFTER THE AFTER

Yo-yoing is the repeated process of weight loss followed by weight gain. This usually happens when you are unable to keep away the weight that you have lost. This may be due to a faulty diet pattern that alternates drastic dieting with sudden binges. New mothers are especially susceptible as lifestyle changes and added responsibilities can give rise to mood swings and make them turn to food for comfort.

What you need to know:

Some studies show that repeated loss and gain of weight can decrease the body's muscle mass and slow down the metabolic rate. The constant yo-yoing of weight can increase stress levels and have a negative psychological effect.

How to deal with it:

✓ Focus on making long-term changes in your diet and physical activity levels. These changes should be easy to handle so that they become a part of your lifestyle. Complicated regimens aren't conducive to new mothers who are struggling to stay on top of their responsibilities. In such cases, more likely than not, their diet will go flying out of the window.

✓ Ensure that your diet isn't too drastic or radical because it will lower your chances of maintaining weight loss and prevent you from the getting the right nutrition. Remember, you are eating for your baby as well.

Fasting

I know, like most dieters, you may be tempted to take this road primarily because of its ability to produce instant, dramatic results. But few realize that this is due to loss of water rather than of body fat. And that, sometime or the other, it will stop giving the same result. The reason is simple: no one can sustain starvation for long periods. Resume eating and all the weight you thought you had lost will be restored. So weight loss due to fasting can never be permanent. Fasting has other side effects. It causes muscles and other tissues to break down and it lowers metabolism. It reduces energy levels and compromises with your immunity. The absence of food can also cause fatigue, irritability, depression and hair fall.

> **Fitness tip**: For sustained weight loss results, regard food not as the foe but as the fuel that drives your body (and as long as you are breastfeeding, that of your baby as well). There is no substitute for a sensible eating plan which nourishes both body and mind.

Feasting

Every time you think your body is responding well to a diet plan, there comes along a wedding, a party, a festival, to ruin it all for you. As if all that were not enough, your baby manages to drive you up the wall and you end up running for cover (and for food). Months of careful eating collapse into an eat-a-thon that will have your weighing scale grunting under excessive weight. It doesn't help that every social event is related in some way to food—birthdays with cakes; parties with unlimited buffets; and festivals with mouth-watering sweets. And when you are faced with so much temptation, how can you keep from giving in?

> **Fitness tip**: Moderation is the key. Limit your intake of festival foods and slightly increase your workout intensity at this time to ensure you don't pile those kilos on back again.

Top Tips to Maintain Weight Loss

⇒ Choose and stick to a lifestyle which combines sensible eating with regular physical activity.

⇒ Eat, don't starve. The focus should be on enjoyable, nutritious meals.

⇒ Don't eliminate, moderate. Enjoy fattening party foods, such as laddoos, karanjis, chaklis and barfis, but in small quantities.

⇒ Make lighter food choices from the spread available for you to eat.

⇒ Avoid large meals.

⇒ Learn to differentiate between hunger and craving.

⇒ Keep yourself active. Exercise will often compensate for once-in-a-while eating sprees and it is better than fasting.

19

Be an Intelligent Shopper

Dear Diary,

Try as I might, I haven't been able to take to vegetables as I really should. If I had my way, I would cook and eat potatoes every day. Still better, I could eat mutton every day. Only today I was looking morosely at the vegetables in my stores and trying desperately to get inspired when I hit upon a novel idea. Why not play on colours? So I decided that today would be a yellow day. So I am cooking a spicy pumpkin dish for dinner. And some moong dal to go with rice. And for dessert, no prizes for guessing, I will be serving sweet limes. ALL YELLOW. It's the same old stuff, only presented differently. It will keep me going for a couple of weeks; then I will have to come up with another idea.

S.

So, what's on your kitchen shelves? Packets of chips, cakes, oily farsans? Then you might as well kiss your dreams of weight loss goodbye. If the foods in your larder are high in calories, that's what's going to end up in your stomach, leaving no space for the essential fruits and vegetables. So I recommend that you learn to replace these diet-unfriendly treats with something more sensible, more conducive to dieting. And for that, you need to turn yourself into an intelligent shopper.

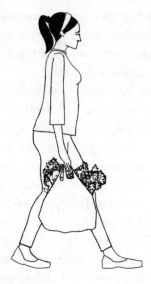

What you need to know:

No matter how rigorous your weightloss plan may be, if temptation is within reach, of course you will grab it.

How to deal with it:

✓ Prepare a list of all the foods which are necessary for your diet and stock up on those. Stick it on your refrigerator door for easy reference.

✓ Of the essentials, you can purchase wholegrain cereals and pulses in bulk. Also store healthy, wholegrain snacks in jars and keep them within easy reach. Fresh fruits and vegetables are best bought fresh daily, though with some smart storing, you can have a week's supply in your refrigerator. For instance, greens, such as methi or lettuce leaves, remain fresh longer if they are cleaned, dried, wrapped in tissue paper and stored in plastic bags. Fresh milk and other dairy products should also feature on your must-have list. If you are a non-vegetarian, make it a point to deep-freeze fish and poultry in smaller portions so that you don't have to take it all out when you need only a little.

✓ If shopping feels like a chore—especially now that you are on baby duty—opt for a service which offers free home delivery of grocery items. But if you are looking for an excuse to get away from the house just for a little while, remember to always shop with a list and never on an empty stomach. Shopping in supermarkets is definitely a test of your will power and there will always be tempting displays of foods which you aren't allowed. So stick to your list and don't go wandering about in the other sections. Also, if you are hungry when shopping, you will be drawn to those cakes and cookies. So go on a full stomach to avoid unnecessary indulgences.

Stock up on:

Green/yellow moongdal	Onions
Brown rice	Apples
Broken wheat (lapsi)	Salad Leaves
Bajre ka atta	Chaatmasala
Jowar ka atta	Basil/Oregano/Rosemary
Wholewheat bread	Coriander and mint leaves
Multigrain bread	Lemons/limes
Rolled oats (oatmeal)	Green/herbal tea
Wholewheat semolina (sooji)	Seasonal fruits
Wholewheat crackers	Tomatoes/Cucumbers
Low-fat tofu	Green leafy vegetables
Low-fat paneer	Spices and herbs
Low-fat yoghurt	Apple cider vinegar
Low-fat feta cheese	Balsamic vinegar
Skimmed milk	Tomato purée

For non-vegetarians

Eggs	Lean fish/Water-packed tuna
Chicken breast (white meat)	Shrimp

Diet no-nos

Ice cream	Deep-fried farsans
Cakes and pastries	Aerated soft drinks
Potato wafers	High-fat cheese
Mayonnaise	Jams/Syrups
Chocolates	Desserts/Puddings

Diet occasionals

Potatoes	Bananas
Peanut butter	Sweet potato
Jackfruit	Mango
Chikoos	Custard apple

Spices unlimited

Lime juice	Green chutney	Cloves
Chaat masala	Green chillies	Cardamoms
Turmeric	Coriander leaves	Cinnamon
Chilli powder	Curry leaves	Pepper
Coriander powder	Mint leaves	Asafoetida
Jeera powder	Tamarind	Bay leaves
Sambar masala	Ginger	Nutmeg
Garam masala	Garlic	Kasuri methi

Top Tips on Stocking

⇒ Use your creativity and use the raw materials in your stock list to create exciting variations in meals. You can take a leaf out of Srishti's book and use colour-coding to spice up your menu.

⇒ The items listed in Diet no-nos are fraught with danger. Keep them out of your kitchen and out of your life.

20

Cooking Smart

Dear Diary,

Some days I miss my mother's cooking. She turns out the simplest of recipes—just a few everyday ingredients thrown together—yet they pack in so much flavour. I still remember tucking into dal, chawal and homemade mango pickle after a hard day's work. Restaurant food was tempting even then, but it lacked the ability to provide comfort and the sense of security that my mother's food did. Everything seemed just right when the whole family got together for dinner. And though I too cook, I fear I don't have the same resourcefulness as my mother, nor are the flavours the same. I should take lessons from her one of these days for I would like to forge the same bond with Mia as she grows up.

S.

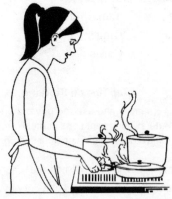

There is nothing quite like home-cooked food. No outside food can quite match it in terms of health and emotional appeal.

What you need to know:

How you cook is as important as *what* you cook. Some cooking methods are healthier and will help you cut out fat and excess calories from foods while retaining their nutritional value. They will help you make delicious yet healthy meals that your child will grow up to appreciate.

How to deal with it:

✓ **Steaming** involves cooking food using steam by placing it in a steamer basket held over boiling water. It does not require oil and helps retain the food's natural flavour, colour and texture. Steam your vegetables in this fashion for a few minutes—until tender but still crisp—to ensure that as many vitamins as possible are retained.

✓ **Pressure-cooking** is effective because it cooks food under steam pressure rather than by adding oil. The process involves trapping steam inside the cooker, allowing the pressure to build up until the temperature rises and drives the steam to cook the food. Pressure-cooking helps preserve nutrients and reduces the cooking time by half.

✓ **Boiling** is cooking food in hot water over a high flame. Again, this does not require oil but it does lead to a loss of water-soluble B and C vitamins. To prevent this, immerse the vegetables in already-boiling water, there by shortening the cooking time and preventing the vitamins from leaching out of the vegetables. Don't discard the water after you are done with it. Use it as vegetable stock for dals, gravies and soups.

✓ **Stir-frying** is similar to sautéing and involves browning foods quickly over high heat in a very small amount of hot oil. High temperatures and constant stirring keep it from sticking and burning. Just ensure that the pan is very hot and shallow and large enough to ensure that the food browns evenly and quickly. The food must be completely dry to prevent it from stewing. Chinese woks or similar pans are wonderful to work with.

✓ **Baking** cooks food in dry heat inside an oven. For this purpose, it takes the water content inside the food and converts it into steam. Of course, it goes without saying that high-calorie and fat-laden cakes and pastries, though baked, are not considered healthy.

Fibre up

Fibre fills you up and sustains you for longer periods. Certain fibre-rich foods, such as flaxseed, bran and wheatgerm, also help stimulate lazy bowels. Be sure to increase water consumption—at least ten glasses a day—for fibre requires ample water to function optimally. More water helps the fibre move more easily through the intestines. To ensure your daily quota of fibre:

✓ Have whole fruits rather than fruit juice. Most of the fibre in fruit is found in the skin, seeds and pulp.

✓ Use a variety of cereals—oatmeal, wholewheat, cornflakes, ragi, jowar, brown rice and barley.

✓ Add vegetables to dishes such as poha or upma. Overcooking reduces the fibre content of vegetables, so steam or cook them until tender but still firm to the bite.

✓ Add a handful of sprouts or sprinkle seeds, such as sesame seeds or flaxseeds, on your cereal.

The fibre content in some foods

Beans and lentils
½ cup cooked lentils	7.8 gm
½ cup cooked kidney beans	7.3 gm
½ cup cooked chickpeas	5.3 gm

Cereals
1 cup cooked oatmeal	4 gm
¾ cup raisin bran	5 gm
¾ cup bran flakes	5 gm

Breads and grains
1 slice wholewheat bread	2 gm
½ cup cooked brown rice	2 gm

Fruits
1 pear with skin	4 gm
1 apple with skin	3.7 gm
1 peach with skin	3.4 gm
2 dried figs	4 gm

Recipes

These are a few of my favourite recipes. Build on these to create your own healthy, diet-friendly cookbook.

1. Strawberry Smoothie

Time taken: 5 min

Serves: 2

Ingredients
1 glass strawberry purée
1 apple, peeled and chopped
1 tsp honey
1 glass skimmed milk

Method:
Blend the ingredients until smooth and drink immediately.

Health score: This refreshing drink packs in vitamins B3, B5, B6, B12, C, E, and biotin, magnesium, manganese, folate, iron, calcium.

2. Fresh Fruits with Honey-Yoghurt Dressing

Time taken: 10 min

Serves: 2

Ingredients
1 large bowl cut fresh fruits (oranges, pears, apples, strawberries)
1 tbsp sunflower seeds
1 tbsp raisins, soaked for ten minutes

For the dressing
½ cup low-fat yoghurt, hung
2 tbsp honey

Method
Mix the fruits, seeds and raisins. Top with the honey-yoghurt dressing and serve.

Health score: Loaded with vitamin E, calcium, potassium, fibre, zinc and protein.

3. High-fibre Cereal

Time taken: 5 min

Serves: 4

Ingredients
8 tbsp oats
2 tbsp sesame seeds, roasted
2 tbsp sunflower seeds
2 tbsp wheat flakes
2 tbsp raisins
2 tbsp chopped almonds
4 tbsp barley flakes or bran
Honey or maple syrup to taste, optional

Method

Mix all the ingredients. Pour skimmed milk over it and serve.

Health score: The cereal packs in vitamins B1, B2, B3, B5, E, and folate, iron, magnesium, selenium, zinc.

4. Legume Spread on Wheat Pita

Soaking time for chickpeas: 6 hours

Preparation time: 15 min

Serves: 4

Ingredients
4 pita breads (or 4 slices of wholegrain bread)
2 tbsp chopped celery
1 tbsp chopped spring onions
2 tbsp chopped peppers (red, green, yellow)
1 tbsp sun-dried tomatoes
Chilli powder, optional
2 tbsp chopped iceberg lettuce

Ingredients for the Legume Spread
250 gm chickpeas
5 tbsp fresh, low-fat yoghurt
Juice of a lemon
2 cloves of garlic, crushed
Salt to taste

Method

Soak the chickpeas for six hours and cook them in a pressure cooker. Cool and drain.

Add the yoghurt, lemon juice, garlic and salt to the chickpeas.

Blend in a blender until smooth. If the mixture is too thick, add water to get the desired consistency.

When serving, add the celery, spring onions, peppers and tomatoes. If you like, add some chilli powder.

To assemble, warm the pita bread, spread the lettuce leaves and top with the chickpea and salad mixture.

Health score: This dish is rich in vitamins B2, B3, B5, B6, C, E, and beta-carotene, folate, iron, lycopene.

5. Oat Banana Cake

Time taken: 15 min

Serves: 4

Ingredients
½ cup oats
½ cup skimmed milk
2 small bananas, mashed
1 cup cottage cheese(paneer), crumbled
3 tbsp unrefined sugar
½ cup raisins, soaked for ten minutes

Method
Boil the oats in milk for five minutes. Cool.

Add the rest of the ingredients to make dough.

Heat the oven and bake for ten minutes. Let cool and serve in slices.

Health score: The cake is loaded with vitamins B12, C, E, and folate, iron, protein, flavonoids, potassium, calcium.

6. Rainbow Upma

Time taken: 20 min

Serves: 4

Ingredients
2 cups roasted dalia
1½ cups water
1 tbsp oil
1 tsp mustard seeds
½ inch piece ginger, finely chopped
1 small onion, diced
1 small carrot, diced
½ capsicum, diced
½ cup corn kernels
1 floret cauliflower, diced
¼ cup coriander leaves, finely chopped
1 tbsp lime juice
Salt to taste

Method
Soak the dalia in water for about half an hour.

Heat oil in a pan, add mustard seeds.

When they splutter, add the chopped ginger and onion. Stir for a minute.
Stir in all the remaining vegetables and cook on a low flame until tender.

Drain water from the dalia and add to the cooked vegetables with some salt.

Add 1½ cups of water and cook until it is absorbed.

Sprinkle lime juice on top and toss in the green coriander. Mix well and serve hot.

Health score: This colourful recipe is packed with vitamins C, E, and folate, iron, magnesium, zinc, protein, potassium, calcium.

7. Chicken Delight

Time taken: 45 min

Serves: 4

Ingredients
4 chicken breast halves
½ tsp seasoned salt
1 tsp Italian seasoning
8-10 French beans, julienned
1 small carrot, julienned (or 1 cup shredded carrots)
1 red pepper, julienned
½ cup crumbled cottage cheese
1 cup fresh tomato and garlic sauce

Method
Preheat the oven to 250°C.

Using a knife, carefully butterfly each chicken breast (make a slit through the centre).

Lay them flat on the chopping board and sprinkle with seasoned salt and Italian seasoning. Place 3-4 strips each of the beans, carrots and red peppers. Sprinkle cottage cheese on top.

Roll the chicken breast up and place seam side down in a medium skillet.

Pour the sauce over the chicken and place in the oven. Bake for 20-25 minutes, basting with the sauce halfway through cooking.

Remove the breasts from the pan.

To serve, slice each breast into 4-5 pieces and arrange in a fan shape. Pour a little extra sauce on the side.

Health score: This dish is rich in vitamins A, K, D, B12, and protein, riboflavin, niacin, calcium.

8. Stir-fry Salad

Time taken: 15 min

Serves: 4

Ingredients
1 tsp oil
1 tsp onion seeds (kalonji)
1 cup capsicum, cut into thin strips
1 spring onion, sliced
½ cup baby corn, sliced
½ cup broccoli florets
½ cup cucumber, sliced
¼ cup bean sprouts
1 small tomato, deseeded and sliced
Salt to taste
1 cup cottage cheese, cut into strips

Method
Heat the oil and add the onion seeds.

Add all the vegetables and salt and sauté on a high flame till tender.

Add the cottage cheese and sauté for another minute.

Remove from heat and serve immediately.

Health score: This one promises the goodness of vitamins A, C and fibre, iron, calcium.

Top Tips to Keep It Healthy

⇒ Consider these options for healthy snacking:

⇒ Wraps: Roll up cottage cheese, vegetables and spreads in a roti for a wholesome bite.

⇒ Sandwiches: There are many toppings to choose from—lettuce, tomato, cucumber, sprouts, cottage cheese or tofu, chicken, fish.Make a different sandwich each day of the week.

⇒ Chaat: Few women can resist the lure of chaat. Give it a healthy spin by adding crunchy moong sprouts, cucumbers, baked sev and a rich tamarind-date chutney.

Dear Diary,

Sometimes, I think I know it all. Other times, I am downright confused and don't know right from wrong. And to think it seems simple enough: eat less to lose more weight. So why should there be so many speed breakers along the way?

S.

The road to weight loss is often bumpy and can throw up quite a few shockers that are capable of derailing your best intentions. Here are a few issues that bother weight-watchers and my suggestions for dealing with them.

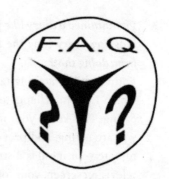

1. **Weight loss techniques have never worked on me before. Why would they work now?**

   Just because something didn't work earlier doesn't mean it won't do so in the future. Maybe you are approaching the problem all wrong. Go in with a defeatist attitude and you've lost the battle even before you've begun. Instead:

☞ Surround yourself with positive affirmations. 'I will lose weight for sure.' 'Nothing is going to stop me this time.' Keep repeating them until they become a sort of mantra for you. They will give you just the confidence boost you need.

☞ Give your goals a reality check. Are you being practical as far as your goals are concerned? Maybe you are aiming to lose too much too soon. Think small at first. Take baby steps. And slowly build up on them.

☞ Don't focus too much on the problem. Channel your energy on finding out solutions. 'I was supposed to lose a pound this week, but I didn't. Maybe it was due to the weekend binge I went on. Okay, so I will keep my portions small, exercise regularly and steel my mind to stick to the diet in the coming week.' That's how it should go.

2. *I maintained a diary like you told me to, and I realized I was bingeing every time the television was on. How do I keep from doing that?*

Eating while watching television breaks an important rule which I tell my clients to follow—focus on your food while eating. This keeps your mind alert as to *what* and *how much* you are eating, and prevents you from overindulging. The minute your mind is distracted by what's happening on the television screen, your food awareness goes out the window. Here are a few pointers to help you with the problem:

☞ If you are at the movies and love popcorn, choose one which is not buttered. And skip the jumbo tub. Stick to the smallest size available.

☞ If you are looking forward to an interesting movie on television, try and have a healthy snack before show time. It will fill your stomach and not make you feel peckish.

☞ Instead of having something to munch on, sip green tea or lime juice—it will give you something to do without adding too many calories.

☞ Try and cut down on television time. Being inactive for long hours in front of the television screen isn't going to take you towards your weight loss goals.

3. *When I see all the good food at parties I can't help myself.*
I've mentioned before that when you are faced with a wide, delicious menu, stick to the one thing you like the most and have that in moderation. There is no sense in wanting to sample everything on offer. Here are some other things which you can try out:

☞ Try and have a healthy snack before you arrive at the party. That way, you won't be very hungry and dying to attack the buffet table.

☞ Fill up on soup and salad to begin with, leaving just enough space for that one sinful treat which you've chosen from among the varied spread.

☞ Eat slowly. The more quickly your plate becomes empty, the more trips to the buffet table you will make.

☞ Stand as far away from the table as possible. You don't want to make it too easy to give in to the temptation.

4. *My baby keeps me awake for the greater part of the night and I find myself sneaking in snacks at unearthly hours.*
Late-night snacks are calorie-monsters and will ruin what is otherwise a perfectly good diet. Here are a few cheat codes:

☞ Have pictures of a slim you pasted on your fridge and

other snack shelves. Looking at them will put you off snack raids.

☞ If you can't sleep, read. Or catch a movie on your DVD player. Listen to music. If you have a 4 a.m. friend, talk to her—anything that will keep your mind off food.

☞ Don't keep fried, unhealthy snacks at hand. You can't eat them if they are not there in the first place.

☞ Finally, ensure that you are eating enough during the day. If you are not, it may explain why you feel ravenous at night. Refer to the chapters *Eating Right* and *Eat Little, Eat Often* to make sure you are on the right track.

5.   *I eat to escape my emotions.*

Motherhood is a melting pot of emotions and most mothers take to eating as a way of seeking comfort. It can wreak havoc on their diet and it is essential that they grow out of that phase. To do that:

☞ Seek other forms of comfort. Get a hobby. Surround yourself with friends. Start a diary.

☞ Keep yourself engaged. Do the household chores. Go grocery-shopping. Exercise. If you are busy, you are less likely to feel like an emotional wreck and less likely to reach out for something to eat.

☞ Don't stock calorie-rich comfort foods, such as cream cookies, mithai, fried farsans and tubs of ice cream or kulfi at home.

6.   *I find it difficult to bounce back after a lapse. I think, after all, what's the point for I know it will happen again?*

It is necessary not to accept a lapse as defeat. It is a slip-up and it happens. What is important is your ability to pick up the pieces and start afresh. Wallowing in guilt for something you failed to do will only lead to more lapses. Learn to accept it as a weak moment and move on with determination and enthusiasm.

7. **Is tofu really good for vegetarians? What is it actually?**
    Tofu is derived from soya bean. It is produced by grinding cooked soya beans so they release a milky substance that is then solidified. It is also known as soya bean curd. Tofu is high in protein, low in saturated fats and is cholesterol-free. Calorie-wise, 100 gm of tofu contains only 73 calories. But do read the label, for soft tofu tends to be higher in fat content than firm tofu. You can use it as a substitute for paneer in sweet or savoury dishes. Most supermarkets stock tofu.

8. **Is it okay to eat mutton every day? I love it.**
    Mutton and pork are full of cholesterol and hidden fat and should be eaten sparingly. Substitute them with lean chicken and fish.

9. **Is rice really the health hazard it is made out to be?**
    Eat rice by all means, but in moderation. Try the unrefined versions—brown rice, red rice, wild rice—they are more filling and contain more fibre.

Take it from me: If you look at it correctly, watching what you eat is the easiest thing in the world. If you look at it differently, it can be the most difficult. The only thing which can keep you going is your resolution to get back into shape. Think about it this way. It's good not only for you but also for your baby, in the sense that it will lift your flagging spirits and boost your self-esteem by making you look and feel good. Certainly a plus for someone who is trying to bring up a baby, what do you say?

SECTION FOUR

EXERCISE

Admit it! You were hoping, now that the baby is born, you would automatically be left with a trimmer figure. Not so. As you survey the scene of all the recent action, you realize many things—your mid-torso crisis is far from over; the tummy continues to look flabby; gone are your well-sculpted abs; the perineal area feels all stretched and sore, and your joints seem just too fragile to do their job. Dancing to your baby's tune all day long isn't helping, either. Nor is the fact that you have no time—and frankly, no energy—to whip yourself into shape. So, should you just leave it to the benevolence of your genes and metabolism to help you bounce back into shape (though this does not always guarantee results)? I'd say not! I'd rather you took matters into your own hands and worked towards revealing the trim you that is lying trapped between the layers of flab and the folds of your skin, but by using my favourite mantra: Slowly and Steadily!

This section is designed to ease you back into the exercise mode. Of course, circumstances are difficult. There really *is* a shortage of time. And you aren't exactly brimming with vigour. Still, if you are sufficiently committed, there are always ways to beat the odds and to sneak in some exercise without making large investments of time (and sometimes, without your even realizing it). This will not only help you move closer to your physical goals but also give you the endorphin boost to stay happy and strong in the face of the many demands of new parenthood.

There are other benefits too:

Improved stamina: Instead of tiring you out, exercise will actually build up your stamina and help you tackle your daily chores with greater energy and efficiency.

Sound sleep: You may argue that there's hardly any time for it, but there's no denying that you will enjoy better quality sleep even if it is just a catnap!

That happy feeling: Courtesy those stress-busting endorphins about which I am always talking.

Looking good: You are bound to feel good about yourself, merely knowing that you are working on your body. In the long run, it will also reward you with a fitter, more slender you!

Stronger muscles: Exercise helps overcome muscle stiffness, makes them less prone to aches and pains, and tones them.

Active bowels: Regular exercise aids the elimination process— just as important a factor as following a healthy diet.

I will take you through some simple moves that you can practise in the initial six weeks of recovery, and then move on to a more comprehensive plan which is serious enough to get you back in shape. Of course, no matter which fitness plan you take up, it is always best to take your doctor into confidence about it and get his go-ahead signal. That done, it is, on your marks, get set, EXERCISE!

22

Slow and Steady

Dear Diary,

Sometimes I think our generation loves making mountains out of molehills. My grandmother bore four children. And she did it without getting into a sweat. She had no need for 'exercise and other silliness' as she labelled it. To be sure, she was not svelte like so many of our film heroines. But she wasn't fat either. Just strong. As an ox. Kind of makes you think, doesn't it? I have only a single kid, yet I find it overwhelming at times. And while I keep cribbing about not losing all the 'baby fat' quickly enough, I am not doing anything about it either. I wish I had my grandmother's spirit. To keep going. No matter what!

S.

The older generation was certainly a hardy lot. But then, they had a hard life that demanded a lot of physical work. Our lives are much easier, more sedentary and require no back-breaking labour. On the other hand, we find ourselves chained to our desks and chairs. The only thing that moves is our finger on the mouse, and a million global transactions are made. Since our jobs won't do our calorie-burning for us anymore, we need exercise to do it. Srishti's grandmother didn't need to work on her abs but you will have to, in order to lose all the 'baby fat' from your pregnancy.

What you need to know:

✓   Too little exercise isn't effective. Too much can be harmful.
✓   Consistent exercise is the key if you want to see results.
✓   It is necessary to monitor the intensity of your exercise to ensure you aren't overdoing it.
✓   Rest periods are as important as workouts.
✓   You need to listen to your body for cues which tell you when to stop.

How to deal with it:

✓   The threshold for exercise tolerance will differ from one new mother to another. Unless recommended otherwise by your gynaecologist, I recommend that you ease into the exercise mode with thirty-minute walks in the beginning. If you can tolerate that comfortably, you may add five–ten minutes per week, and slowly build up the duration to an hour.
✓   After the first six weeks, you should exercise daily but if that sounds like too much at first, begin with three days a week. In my postnatal exercise classes, I introduce enough variety each day to keep things interesting and to give specific muscles time to recover. Since every regimen should include exercises that build stamina, strength and suppleness (refer to the next chapter for details) and also encourage the practice of deep breathing and relaxation, an ideal plan would be:

i.   Walking/swimming/aqua aerobics/cycling: three–five days a week

ii. Yoga/stretching/strength training: two–three days a week

iii. Deep breathing and relaxation: seven days a week

Of course, how consistently you can exercise will depend on health considerations. That is why it is best to consult your doctor while drawing up a plan.

✓ The talk test is an effective indicator of intensity. A low-to-moderate pace (ideal in your just-delivered condition) is one that lets you carry on a light conversation but not sing when exercising. Once your body settles down to this pace, you can turn up the intensity a few more notches. At high intensity, even speech will become difficult.

✓ Allow up to twenty-four hours of rest for your worked-out muscles. To allow them to overcome exhaustion, train with weights every other day rather than daily.

✓ Given the stress and strain through which your body has just gone, it is important that you don't add to its burden. So watch out for the following signs—pain, cramps, light-headedness, dizziness—and if you detect any one of these, stop. If the symptoms persist, consult your doctor immediately.

If you have stayed physically active during your pregnancy, it will have helped you maintain your stamina, strength and muscle tone. It will also have prepared you for the hard work of labour, and made it easier for you, after the delivery, to bounce back to your pre-pregnancy weight and figure.

Continue your exercise afterwards to get back in shape, lose weight and improve stamina to cope with the new pressures. There are usually no exercise restrictions, post-baby, unless you have some medical concerns. Even if you haven't exercised during pregnancy, it is not too late! For, NOW is the time to be concentrating on your present and future, and on finding healthy ways to stay fit and fabulous.

23

The Three Pillars of Fitness

Dear Diary,

Up to now, my idea of fitness entailed one of three things—walking, jogging or running on the treadmill at the gym. If I did one of these regularly, I would be doing enough, or so I thought. But Namita told me that these three exercises constituted just one aspect of exercise, that is building stamina. However, there were two others that were just as important—building strength and increasing suppleness. Together— stamina, strength and suppleness—they are hard to beat. She promised she would help me draw a fitness plan that would incorporate all three in my next session and I am eagerly looking forward to it.

All pumped up,
S.

Most people I know follow a one-dimensional workout. There are many who, like Srishti, are content with just cardio. Their workout consists of putting on shoes, plugging in earphones for music and going through the paces on the jogging track. Then there are others, mainly guys, who prefer to pump iron in gyms. They spend all their time heaving and straining with weights in their attempt to build bodies à la Salman Khan. Neither party thinks much of the other's workout. What neither realizes is just how much more effective their exercise would be if they combined both kinds—cardio and weights. Throw in one more element—stretches—and their fitness targets would be well within easy reach. And this stands for new mothers too!

What you need to know:

1.   Any exercise plan must address three important issues:

i.   **Cardiovascular fitness**

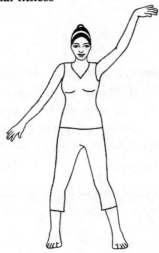

It conditions your heart and enables it to function more effectively. It contributes to the first 's' of fitness—*stamina*. Stamina is your body's ability to sustain physical activity for prolonged periods. It is built by any movement which is rhythmic and continuous, such as walking, and uses the large muscle groups in your body.

ii.   **Strength training**
It improves muscle mass and power, makes your bones stronger,

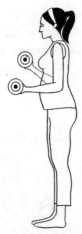

and keeps your joints in good working condition. It is responsible for the second 's' of fitness—*strength*. A good indicator of your strength is the ease with which you can undertake daily activities, such as standing, sitting, and lifting heavy bags. One can use body weight, light weights, resistance bands or exercise machines to build strength.

> **Did you know?** Strength training improves calcium absorption in the body, giving you stronger bones.

iii. Flexibility

It ensures that your body remains agile and less vulnerable to muscle stress. It makes up the third 's' of fitness—*suppleness*. Suppleness helps your body go through a wide range of motions, such as bending and stretching, without breaking into a sweat. It is as much a part of your everyday life as stamina and strength. Flexibility is built by stretches which create a slight degree of tension, but without physical discomfort, which is especially desirable in view of the fact that your body is already a bit sore from the trauma of delivery.

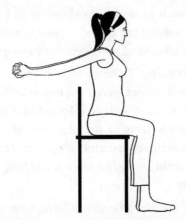

2. No exercise routine is complete without a warm-up and a cool-down. They might appear to be a waste of precious time but they can actually protect you from soreness and injury.

    Warm-up is a way of preparing your body for a workout. It increases your heart rate gradually, boosts circulation and improves muscle elasticity.

    Cool-down is a kind of signal to your body that your workout is coming to an end. If you stop exercising abruptly, it shocks your body and this can cause light-headedness, cramps or soreness. Instead, you gradually draw it to a close. A cool-down enables your body to recover, repair and regenerate itself effectively after a workout.

How to deal with it:

✓ To ensure that your regimen is well-rounded and comprehensive, you should include the following:

   Cardiovascular fitness: To keep your heart pumping, set aside thirty to sixty minutes every day of the week for exercises, such as walking, swimming and cycling. (More details on walking are provided later in the chapter.) This will benefit your lungs and circulatory system as well.

Strength training: It must address every major muscle group, to be done not more than two to three times a week, and not on successive days. (More details on working out at home follow later in the chapter.) The breaks are to allow the muscles to rest and recuperate. Added benefits of strength training include a more toned body and increased metabolism.

Flexibility: Practise an exercise form, such as yoga, at least three times a week. Added benefits include improved blood and nutrient flow to the joints, relaxed muscles and better posture. For best results, hold each stretch for at least ten to thirty seconds.

✓ To acclimatize your body before and after the workout, do the following:

Warm-up: Before immersing yourself in your exercise regimen spend five to ten minutes walking or spot-marching.

Cool-down: Taper off activity in both intensity and pace to allow your body to drop into its pre-exercise level gradually.

Note: Consult your doctor before you embark on any exercise routine.

Take a walk

If you ask me, it is the easiest thing to do simply because it doesn't make too many demands on your body. And, having just delivered a baby, you will admit that that can be a boon.

So as soon as you are able, put on your shoes and take a walk. This low-impact cardio activity will give your heart, lungs and bones a complete workout without putting too much strain on your joints. But just because walking is easy doesn't mean there is no technique to it. The better your form is while walking, the more benefits you will gain from it. Here's how to walk the perfect walk:

✓ Hold yourself straight, keep your head centred between your shoulders and push your chest out a bit.
✓ Bend your elbows and propel your arms backwards and forwards in tandem with your legs.
✓ Keep your abs tucked in.
✓ Your feet should be placed firmly on the ground. As you take a step forward, strike first with your heel and then press down your full foot on to the ball of your foot, and now, you are ready to take the next step.

I keep telling my clients that walking can contribute a lot to keeping them from getting bored. Since no fixed venue is needed, you can skip the neighbourhood jogging track and try the city garden instead. Nothing is more rejuvenating than walking surrounded by nature. The highlight of Srishti's day was walking on the lawns of her residential complex garden. As she confided in me, she found it soothing and very relaxing. Just the antidote for frazzled nerves! You can also try changing the pace. Get a friend to accompany you and to set the pace; the change in speed will keep you occupied. If you reach a point where you are looking for something more challenging, try an uphill walk. It can be very demanding, so make sure you've built up your stamina first by undertaking regular walks.

Dos and Don'ts

⇒ As I have mentioned before, maintain the right posture when you are walking.
⇒ For it to make a difference, walk at a pace that lets you talk but not sing.
⇒ Never use hand or ankle weights when walking for they will increase risk of injury.
⇒ Always stretch after your walk. The calf stretch and the front and back of the thigh stretches are particularly useful (Refer to the section titled *Go Stretch*).

Weight and Watch

By strengthening your muscles, you can reduce the risk of injury which may result from constantly handling the baby and also lessen the backache.

Things you will need

✓ Dumb-bells or two 500 ml bottles filled with water
✓ A mat or a carpet
✓ A chair

1. **Wall Push-ups**—For a great upper body

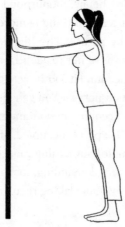

Stand with your face towards the wall. Your body should be parallel to it. Keeping your back straight (do not slouch or arch your back), place your palms flat on the wall, shoulder-width apart. Bend your elbows as you lean forward towards the wall, then return to the starting position. Repeat sixteen times.

2. **Single-arm Row**—For strengthening the back and improving the posture

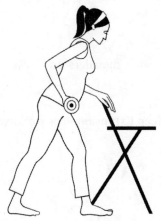

Place your left hand on the back of a chair for support. Lean forward so that your body is diagonal to the floor. Hold a dumb-bell in your right hand and, bending it at the elbow, lift it towards your waist. Lower and repeat for sixteen counts. Then change your arm and repeat the sequence.

3. **Bicep Curl**—For adding strength and definition to your biceps
    Hold dumb-bells in both hands, palms facing upwards. Bending the elbows, tense your biceps and lift the dumb-

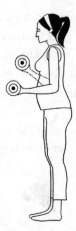

bells towards your shoulders and lower. Repeat sixteen
times.

4. **Overhead Tricep Extension**—For working the back of the
    arms

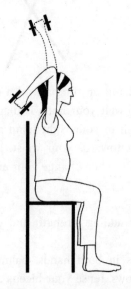

Sit on the edge of a chair, back erect. Holding one dumb-bell in both hands, raise your arms overhead. Now bend them at the elbows, bringing the dumb-bell down behind your head, and return to the starting position. Repeat sixteen times.

5. **Lateral Shoulder Raise**—For toning shoulders to create a well-sculpted look

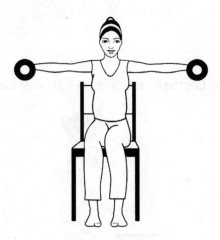

Sit on a chair, arms hanging down at the sides, holding a weight in each hand, elbows slightly curved forward. Raise arms until elbows are shoulder height. Lower arms, and return to the starting position. Repeat sixteen times.

6. **Calf Raise**—For toning the calves
Stand with your shoulders pushed back, chest raised. Raise your heels as high as you can so that you are standing on the tips of your toes. Lower them and repeat sixteen times.

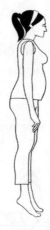

7. **Standing Leg Extension**—For strengthening the thighs

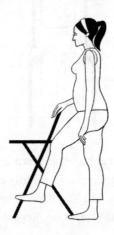

Stand tall. Holding the back of a chair for balance, lift your left leg, bending your knee. Now extend this leg from the knee. Repeat sixteen times, then repeat with the right leg.

8. **Standing Pelvic Tilt**—For strengthening the back, hips and abs

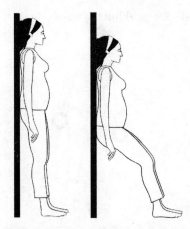

Stand with your back to a wall, feet placed shoulder-width apart, heels away from the wall. Press the small of your back flat against the wall and slide down an inch or two, bending the knees slightly. Hold for ten seconds and then return to the starting position. Repeat twelve to sixteen times.

9. **Side-position Leg Lift**—For exercising the outer thighs and hips

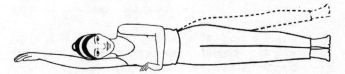

Lie down on one side; stretch your arm out under your head. Slowly raise the upper leg so that it is higher than your hips. Bring it down slowly. Repeat sixteen times with each leg. Avoid tilting your chin to your chest when you are lifting your leg; to protect your neck from undue strain, let your arm support your head.

10. **Waist Bend**—For working the waist

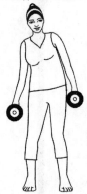

Stand with one dumb-bell in each hand. From the waist, lean to the right, then return to the starting position. Repeat sixteen times, then switch sides. Keep your back straight and your abs pulled in when leaning to the side.

Dos and Don'ts

⇒ Let your movements be slow and controlled to avoid injuring joints which have been loosened during pregnancy.

⇒ Focus on getting the technique right. Make it a point to exercise in front of a mirror or get someone to supervise your moves. Using the wrong technique could be more harmful than helpful.

⇒ Create a base before building on it. Begin with lighter weights to prevent muscle soreness. As you grow more confident, you can add to the weights.

⇒ Listen to your body. If a particular exercise causes pain or discomfort, discontinue it. Consult your gynaecologist if the pain persists.

⇒ If a joint is particularly stiff or painful, avoid exercises that will overburden it. In any case, avoid extreme lifts and raises as they can strain your back.

⇒ If you are working out in a gym, stick to machines instead of free weights. They are safer and require less expertise. Even resistance bands are a good option.

Go Stretch

If you are struggling with minor aches, pains and general body stiffness post-delivery, you might want to try these gentle stretches. They are perfect for coaxing your body into becoming agile once more.

> **Tip**: Unless mentioned otherwise, hold each stretch for ten to twenty seconds.

1. **Neck Stretch**

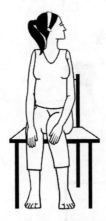

Turn your head to the right side and look over your right shoulder. Hold and return to the starting position. Repeat on the left side.

2. **Shoulder Stretch**
    Cross your left arm over your chest and place your right hand on the left arm just on the elbow, using it to push the right arm higher up on the chest. Switch arms.

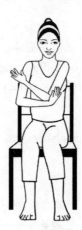

3. **Upper Back Stretch**

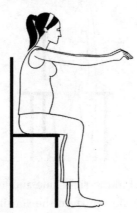

Extend and stretch your hands in front of you and feel the stretch in your upper back.

4. **Chest Stretch**
Sit with a straight back. Extend or clasp your hands behind your back and slowly lift your hands up until you feel a stretch in your chest muscles.

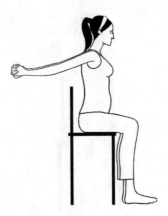

5. **Overhead Arm Stretch**

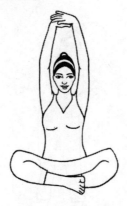

With hands placed one on the other, raise your arms over your head. Now stretch your arms upward until you feel the stretch in your spine and arms.

6. **Shoulder Roll**
Place your fingers on your shoulders, roll the shoulders, first forward and then back. Repeat five times.

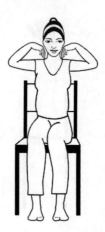

7.   **Waist Stretch**

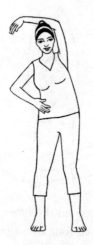

Stand with your feet shoulder-width apart, knees slightly bent, toes pointing straight ahead. Place your right hand on your hip and extend the left hand over your head. Now bend to the right and hold. Repeat on the other side.

8. **Cobbler Stretch**

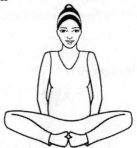

Sit down with your knees bent, soles touching each other. Feel the stretch in your inner thighs. Hold for ten seconds.

9. **Cat–Camel Stretch**

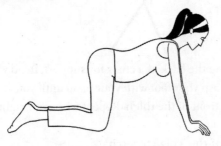

Get down on all fours with your hands directly under your shoulders, and your knees under your hips. Gently arch or curve your back by bringing your belly downwards. Hold for five seconds.

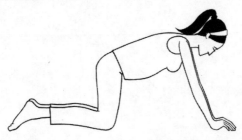

Now arch your back upwards to resemble the hump of a camel. Again hold for five seconds. Repeat both movements seven times.

10. **Front-of-the-Thigh Stretch**

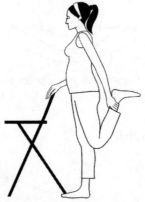

Holding the back of a chair for support, bend your left knee and grasp your foot with your hand until you feel the stretch in the front of the thigh. Repeat with your right leg.

11. **Back-of-the-Thigh Stretch**

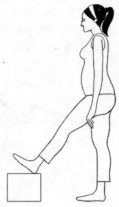

Place one leg on an elevated platform, such as a low wooden stool. Keeping your hips squared, bend forward at the waist. Hold and repeat with the other leg.

12. **Calf Stretch**

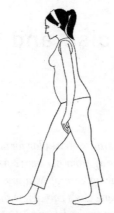

Take a step forward with your right foot. Bend it at the knee, keeping the left leg straight. Now roll your hips forward towards the bent knee, both feet pointing ahead. Both feet should be firmly pressed on the ground. Hold and then change legs.

Dos and Don'ts

⇒ Don't forget to warm up with light cardio before undertaking stretches.
⇒ Stretch in fluid movements, without bouncing or jerking.
⇒ Try and relax when you hold a stretch. Breathe deeply and slowly.
⇒ Do not overextend a stretch until it becomes painful.
⇒ Focus on the part that is being stretched. Feel the stretch.
⇒ It is best to work on stretches after an intense workout. Since your muscles are already warmed up, there is less risk of injury. Besides, stretching is calming and relaxing and hence, a perfect way to end your workout.

24

Exercise and the Baby

Dear Diary,

When Namita came up with an exercise plan for me, I was apprehensive. Would that mean time away from my baby? As a new mother I am overly obsessive about taking care of Mia myself. I cannot imagine surrendering her to someone else's care. How then would I be able to concentrate on the workout she had drawn up? Namita explained that it wasn't wrong to spend some time away from the baby. In fact, it was essential for my own well-being. But, she said, just in case I was not convinced and knowing that this would give me the perfect excuse not to exercise, she had already incorporated moves that would allow Mia to participate. What! Mia help me in my workout? How was that possible?

S.

Yes, it is. In fact, some fitness classes encourage new mothers to bring their babies along for an interactive workout. This not only creates a stronger bond between mother and child but also allows new mothers to seek comfort in others like them. But that comes much later. In the first six weeks, it is necessary to concentrate on those body parts that need immediate attention, specifically the stomach, the abs and the pelvic region. In this chapter, I will list out exercises which you can begin performing almost immediately.

And then, when your workout grows more structured, more serious, I'll suggest everyday exercises with a twist that will enable your darling to help you in your quest to burn those calories.

What you need to know:

0–6 Weeks

✓ The abdomen and the pelvic region are the most affected during pregnancy and delivery, and they benefit from immediate attention and exercise.

✓ From the second week onwards after delivery, I advise my clients to start walking for exercise. Resuming exercise early helps overcome problems such as urinary incontinence more quickly.

After Six Weeks

✓ Now you can start considering a more structured, serious exercise regimen to get back in shape.

✓ Don't expect instantaneous results. I'd say give it a year to achieve your final target. Pushing your body too hard to get there more quickly is more harmful than helpful.

How to deal with it:

0–6 Weeks

1. **Kegel**, **pelvic tilt** and **abdominal compressions** target the main problem areas and can be undertaken within twenty-four hours after delivery. Spend just five to ten minutes on these exercises:

    i. **Kegel**: Lie down on your back, bend your knees, raise the pelvis and squeeze the muscles as if to stop the flow of urine. Make sure not to contract the muscles in your stomach as you do this. Hold for five to ten seconds, then release.

ii. **Pelvic tilt**: Stand with your back to the wall, feet placed shoulder-width apart, and heels a few inches away from the wall. Press the small of your back flat against the wall and slide down an inch or two. Hold for ten seconds and then return to the starting position. In the other version, lie down on your back with knees bent; tilt your pelvis by drawing the tailbone up and pressing the back down while pulling in the abdominal muscles. Hold the position for five to ten seconds and release.

iii. **Abdominal compression**: These should be done preferably lying down. Take a deep breath and let your belly expand. Relax and exhale, contracting your stomach by pulling in your belly button as far as you can towards the spine. Do this ten times.

2. When it comes to walking, it is necessary to take baby steps. Start with ten minutes and slowly build it up five minutes at a time. (Refer to the chapter above for tips on proper posture while walking.) If done right, walking will help strengthen your lower body and improve your posture as well.

After Six Weeks

✓ Concentrate on an exercise regimen which focuses on the three parameters discussed in the previous chapter: cardiovascular fitness, strength training and flexibility.

✓ The regimen should be comprehensive but comfortable.

✓ Ask yourself the following questions to ensure you aren't overdoing it:

i. Is your workout leaving you feeling fatigued? Exercise should energize, not drain. If it is draining you, you need to tone it down.

ii.   Is it causing pain or bleeding? If it is, stop exercising and consult your doctor.

iii. Are you getting enough rest? Allowing your body to relax is just as important as getting enough exercise.

iv.   Is your urine clear? Breastfeeding mothers need to stay hydrated and since exercise can further deplete the water reserves in your body, you need to drink up.

v.   Is your baby's appetite waning? High-intensity exercise could cause excessive lactic acid build-up in your body. Some of it gets absorbed into your milk giving it a sour taste that can put your baby off. As mentioned in the chapter on *Breastfeeding and Lactation*, you could try feeding him before exercise or an hour or two after.

Exercising with the baby

Having a baby is no reason not to exercise. In fact, there are many fun ways in which you can make your baby a part of your exercise regimen:

1.   **Walking**

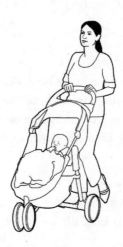

Find a stroller that is light, durable and moves easily, and you are all set to go. Taking your baby along for a walk kills two birds with one stone—you get to exercise as well as spend quality time with your darling. If you like company, plan a foursome with another new mother.

2. **Wall Squat with Baby**
Holding your baby, stand with your back pressed against the wall, feet shoulder-width apart and heels a few inches away from the wall. Slide down to a squat so that your thighs are parallel to the ground. Hold for three seconds and return to the starting position. Repeat twelve times.

3. **Abdominal Curl with Baby**

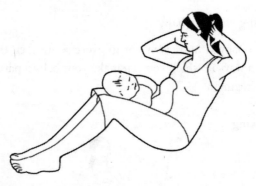

Lie down on the floor, knees bent. Place your baby against your thighs ensuring that his head and back are supported. Now using your abs, try and come up until your shoulders are lifted off the floor. Go down again and relax. Repeat twelve times.

4. **Bridge with Baby**
Lie down on a mat, knees bent. Rest the baby against your thighs. Do a Kegeland, lift your hips and lower back off

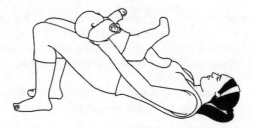

the floor. Return to the starting position and relax. Repeat twelve times.

5. **Chest Press with Baby**

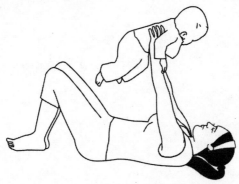

Lie down on a mat, knees bent. Hold the baby on your chest. Extend your arms and lift up the baby (please ensure that your baby can support its head when you do this). Return to the starting position and relax. Repeat twelve times.

Dos and Don'ts

⇒ Listen to your body. Your decision to exercise should depend on how your body is coping with the aftermath of delivery.

⇒ Keep it slow and simple at first. As I keep telling my clients, there is no point trying to bite off more than you can chew. At this point in your life, you need exercise which strengthens your body without overburdening it.

⇒ If something hurts, stop exercising immediately. It is best to consult your doctor if the pain persists.
⇒ Don't make excuses. If you can't go outdoors on a certain day, try and exercise at home. If you don't have an hour to spare, try thirty minutes.
⇒ Make exercise a part of your daily routine. It should feature in your to-do plan for the day, every day.

25
Time Crunch

Dear Diary,

With Namita there can be no excuses. Just yesterday she took me to task for not sticking to my fitness regimen. Why doesn't she understand that sometimes it just isn't possible to take time out for it? In any case, a whole hour of exercise is just too much. That's all the free time I get in a day. If I use it to exercise, when do I sleep? Or watch television? Or do something that's relaxing?

Grumpily,
S.

I must have heard this one a hundred times: 'We'd love to exercise but where is the time?' To be fair, I realize that no one has it tougher than new mothers who are saddled with a responsibility which takes up most of their waking hours. But desperate times call for desperate measures. And if you are serious about getting back into shape, you must make every nanosecond count. It is no sweat, really. All you need are some techniques or time management that will help you beat the clock.

What you need to know:

✓   Some exercise is better than no exercise.

✓ One of my clients felt so rushed for time that she confided in me: 'I can rest or I can exercise. I cannot do both.' My advice: Rest is as important to physical and emotional well-being as exercise; don't sacrifice one at the altar of the other.

How to deal with it:

✓ If thirty minutes seems too large a chunk for you to keep aside, break your regimen into modules of ten or more minutes. Aim for two fifteen-minute or three ten-minute instalments per day. (Refer to **Exercise on the Run** at the end of this chapter for more details.)

✓ If your household help plays truant, turn your chores into a workout. Feel the stretch as you clean the shelves and swab the floor. Need to buy groceries? That is a good way to stretch your legs by walking up and down the supermarket aisles. Throw in some dance moves when vacuuming.

✓ Invest in exercise equipment—stationary bike, treadmill, resistance bands or free weights. Having these around will enable you to exercise as and when you get some spare time. Also, you will have no excuses *not* to exercise.

✓ Use television time to squeeze in some exercise. Get some stretches done or train with weights as you follow the characters in your favourite soap. Put away the remote and work up a sweat walking up to the screen every time you want to change the channel.

✓ If you've already started working from home, use coffee breaks to burn some calories on the stationary bike. When on the phone, walk as you talk. Take time out from staring at the computer screen to stretch your back, neck, arms and shoulders.

✓ No matter what you are doing, make it a habit to keep your abdomen sucked in.

✓ If you are sitting down or travelling, use the time to work all your muscle groups by contracting and relaxing them. This is good for the circulation.

✓ Take the stairs instead of the elevator every time you need to run errands. It's good cardio and will develop your stamina.

✓ Finally, any time is a good time to relax. Take slow, deep breaths to calm your body and mind.

Exercise on the run

If you have just ten minutes: Go for a walk. If you can't leave the baby, take him with you.

If you have fifteen–twenty minutes: Plan a session that includes Kegels, abdominal contractions, crunches, back extensions and calf lifts.

If you have thirty minutes: Take a walk or use the stationary bike/treadmill for the first fifteen–twenty minutes to get your heart pumping. Then devote the remaining ten–fifteen minutes to stretches and strength training.

26

FAQ

Dear Diary,

Most of my friends are quite taken with Namita. I often quote her nowadays and while I do occasionally grumble about how strict she is, I realize that it is slowly getting me the results I want. And now my friends want her to help them with their own doubts. Well, why not? The next time I meet her, I will be sure to carry a list of some of their queries.

S.

1. **I can't give up food! What to do?**

   Srishti's friend, the one with the twins, admitted she had no control over her diet. She loved food and often sought comfort from it when the stress got too much. She didn't mind exercising as long as she could continue to eat to her heart's content.

   'Would that work?' Srishti asked me.

   No, it wouldn't, I was sorry to say. Exercise is only one half of the solution. It helps you burn fat and tone your body but that alone isn't enough to knock those extra pounds off. To do that you need to monitor your food intake as well. My formula is: 70 per cent diet + 30 per cent exercise =

weight loss. If, like Srishti's friend, you are struggling with your will power, try focusing on your goal. Picture yourself slim once again, as in your pre-pregnancy days. Picture yourself in your old jeans. How about sticking pictures of your old svelte self on the refrigerator? It will put an end to your midnight snack raids for sure. Picture yourself at the receiving end of compliments. These visualizations will help you stay on track with both diet and exercise. As far as stress is concerned, explore other, more creative ways to deal with it. Try your hand at painting. Write poetry. Start gardening. An engaging hobby is just the stress-buster you need and it will keep you from reaching out for that packet of chips. It might seem difficult but in the end it will all have been worth it.

2. *I would really rather starve than exercise. Isn't that much easier?*

Unlike Srishti's other friend, Anita found crash dieting much more rewarding than exercise. It is so much easier *not* to eat than to make that effort to move your body. And it shows great results too, she claimed.

'So why bother to exercise?' was her query.

Crash dieting is never a good idea. Even if it were, how long could you keep it up? Some day or the other, you will give in and how! All the weight you have lost will be regained and you will be back to square one. But that's not the only reason why it is bad. Crash dieting gives you splendid results in the short run but only because of loss of muscle mass. Studies show that in people who diet, about 25 per cent of weight loss is due to loss of muscle mass. In people who exercise and diet, this loss is only about 8 per cent. Exercise prevents loss of muscle and hence it is as necessary as a healthy—not crash—diet. It also increases your metabolism by as much as 25 per cent after a workout.

3. *I feel trimmer but not lighter. What do you think is the problem?*
Naina was in a quandary. After exercising for almost six months after delivery, she felt trimmer, fitter. She was even able to get into some of her pre-pregnancy outfits. But the weighing scale refused to register the change.

'Am I or am I not losing weight?' she wondered.

Losing weight and losing inches are two different things. Exercise alone, as I have said before, helps you shape up but it doesn't help you lose weight. Naina's workouts strengthened bones, melted fat and built muscle mass. They helped her lose inches from her frame but not actual weight. For the weighing scale to register a change, it isn't enough to maintain your calorie intake; you have to bring it down to make a difference.

4. *I am gaining weight despite exercise. How do I lose it?*
In contrast, Laila's weighing scale registered a change just a couple of months after she began exercising to get rid of her pregnancy fat. Only, it was in the opposite direction.

'Why am I exercising and still putting on weight?' she wanted to know.

There are two reasons for it. One, it is normal to feel hungrier when you start exercising because of increased metabolism. But this usually stabilizes over time and stops being an issue. Two (and this seemed to be Laila's case), most people believe that exercise gives them the licence to eat more than usual. This negates any benefits that a combined diet and exercise plan would have on their body. The result—weight gain.

5. *If you stop exercise, the muscles turn to fat. Is that correct?*

Change is the only constant for Chetna. She took it into her head to exercise and did so consistently for a couple of months. Then she tired of it and dropped the idea completely.

'I've heard that if I stop, all the muscle I've built will turn back into fat. So why bother building it up with weights in the first place?' she explained.

This is a common misconception. Fat and muscle are two different things and they are not interchangeable. If you stop exercising, your muscles will go back to their pre-toned state but they cannot turn into fat.

6. *Why do we need weights?*

Jigna considered cardio important above everything else, even weight training. She loved being outdoors, and jogging gave her the perfect excuse to head to the nearest park, a practice she resumed a couple of months after delivery. She loved that it tested her endurance and boosted her stamina.

'Where was the need to fiddle with weights?' she asked me.

Weights build muscle and muscles boost metabolism. The more muscle you have, the faster is your metabolism. Unlike fat, muscle uses more oxygen and calories to maintain itself. Reason enough to do some fiddling, wouldn't you say?

7. *Why is it so difficult to stick to exercise?*

Like all New Year resolutions, Bharati found it hard to keep to her resolve to exercise.

'Why is it so difficult to keep the momentum going?' she complained.

In an attempt to prove a point, most people start themselves on a heavy-duty routine not realizing that they first need to lay a proper foundation for it. It's like pushing yourself to write a novel even before you've learnt to write ABC. So, of course, the attempt ends in failure. Push yourself too hard too soon and it will undermine your confidence and you will find yourself slipping. In the worst scenario, you will end up with injuries or a physical burnout. So, start slow and go steady. If you are aiming for an hour-long run on the jogging track, first start with a half-hour walk. As you grow in confidence, so will your resolve to stick to your routine. Boredom is another reason why people tend to give up. If you've stuck to a routine for a long time, maybe it's time to ring in some changes. If you've always done yoga, you might want to try Pilates for a change. Instead of jogging, you might consider a dance class to burn calories. Remember, if an exercise regimen is not enjoyable, you will find many excuses not to stick to it. Find something which you really enjoy and which is safe and effective, and you will find it easier to keep working at it.

Take it from me: Your body is a machine. If not used, it will rust away. If overworked, it will develop signs of wear and tear. At this critical moment in your life, when all your energy is concentrated on caring for your newborn, you need to find the right balance between rest and exercise for optimum results. To exercise with some consistency, you need to stay motivated. Here are a few tips to stay on top of the game:

Take baby steps: Starting small allows you to grow in confidence and stamina.

Seek company: Having an exercise buddy keeps you from getting bored.

Turn on the music: Jazz up your workout with your favourite tunes.

Keep it varied: Keep introducing new moves, new forms of exercise, to keep your interest going.

Take rest: It helps your body recuperate and stay in top form.

COMMON CONCERNS

'I have such-and-such a problem. Why is that? What can I do about it?'

'My friend suffered from this medical condition after delivery. Do I have it too?'

'Am I really depressed? Should I tell my doctor? Or am I just blowing it out of proportion?' These and many other questions may have crossed your mind. And though there is no dearth of information these days, not all of it is correct or even relevant. Keeping this in view, I've designed this section to explore some common concerns that mothers may face after delivery. It attempts to explain these concerns as succinctly as possible and suggests ways to manage them.

27

Sleep Deprivation

Dear Diary,

In my younger days, I remember, my friends and I would make bets about staying up all night to watch movies during the summer holidays. I never had the stamina for it and would fall asleep almost immediately. Needless to say, I lost every time. How I wish I could make the same bet now! For, even if I want to fall asleep, I know I can't. Mia keeps strange timings—she is awake for the greater part of the night and her feeding schedule is such that I end up wide awake all night long. The daytime isn't much different and I manage not more than a few winks at a time. They are hardly enough and, as a result, my brain is beginning to get woolly—do you know, yesterday, I forgot where I had kept Mia's freshly laundered cloth diapers? That's until my mother extracted them from the fridge where I must have mistakenly stowed them, all nice and crisply cold.

Distracted and dazed,
S.

It's ironic, isn't it? Sleep, the very thing that could possibly keep you relaxed, rejuvenated and raring to meet your baby's umpteen demands, is denied to you in the initial months immediately after delivery. How are you supposed to take care of your baby when you haven't had a decent night's sleep in a while? How are you supposed to enjoy moments with your baby and take delight in every new trick that he learns, while your body and mind are screaming for some serious shut-eye? A lack of sleep can cause serious problems, including post-partum depression in some mothers. The solution? If you ask me, use all the help you can get to bring up your baby. There's no merit in wanting to do it all alone. Second, learn to snatch precious moments from your hectic schedule for a quick nap no matter what time of day it is. A well-rested mother makes a better mother, I say.

What you need to know:

✓ Brand-new mothers are often bewildered by the sleep pattern of their babies. They sleep often but in short bouts (ranging from half an hour to about three–four hours) which are punctuated by feeding. In keeping with this haphazard schedule, your baby may sleep throughout the day and stay up for the larger part of the night—and you have no option but to follow suit.

✓ Newborns aren't cued into day and night and it takes them a while to learn—much to the dismay of their sleep-deprived mothers—that night time is for sleeping. Some studies indicate that new mothers may have to wait about three to five months before they can hope that their baby, along with themselves, get a decent night's sleep.

✓ For most of the time that they spend sleeping, babies are in the active sleep mode; signs include fluttering eyelids, irregular breathing, making sounds or moving a little. This makes them light sleepers and prone to waking up at the slightest disturbance.

How to deal with it:

For the baby:

✓ Make it easy for your baby to distinguish between day and night by monitoring lighting patterns—keep it bright during the day, dimmed at night. Involve the baby in your daily chores during the day and slowly fade out activity by nightfall. It's your way of telling him the day is winding down and it is time to retire for the night.

✓ Keep it quiet during night-time feedings. Chances are that the baby will feed and go right back to sleep. If you create too much of a racket—put on lights, make a noise, move yourself and the baby too much—you risk waking him up totally. Putting him back to sleep in this case will take much longer.

✓ Try massages. Studies show that they may improve your baby's sleep pattern. Just make sure the masseuse is qualified to give infant massages. And why not get one yourself? It may be just the thing to ease your stress and make you feel relaxed.

✓ Breastfeed him just before bedtime and for longer than usual. Breast milk contains tryptophan which helps manufacture melatonin, a hormone responsible for inducing drowsiness. A larger meal ensures that your baby will sleep for a longer time.

✓ To ensure he isn't disturbed once he is asleep, avoid moving him for about half an hour (even if he has fallen asleep in your arms) during which time he will move from the active mode and settle comfortably into deep sleep.

For yourself:

✓ Eat right—calmly and slowly. Rushing through your food will upset your digestion and cause you sleepless nights.

Even the quantity of food matters—eat too much and you will be worried about facing the weighing scale the next morning; eat too little and you will be craving a midnight snack. Both will affect your sleep.

✓ Create the right ambience for sleep. Invest in a good mattress—one that is firm yet soft on your back. Have a hot bath and a glass of milk before you retire for the night. Stay off caffeine closer to your bedtime and avoid too many liquids unless you want to make frequent bathroom trips in the middle of the night.

✓ Learn to relax. Take a deep breath and feel all your worries stream out as you exhale. Do things that improve your mood. Listen to some music. No matter what you do, don't take your anxieties to bed with you for you will only end up tossing and turning all night.

✓ Exercise daily. It busts stress and makes you feel good about yourself. It also induces tiredness and sleep.

28

Abdominal Separation (Diastasis Recti)

Dear Diary,

My friend with the twins came over yesterday and we got around to talking about medical conditions. It seems she has dia something or the other—it means there is a gap in her abdomen. Did I have it? It was easy to find out, she said, and soon I was lying down on my back and she had her finger pressed into my skin somewhere below my belly button. You don't, she said with the air of one who knows it all. I didn't trust her diagnosis so I asked my doctor about it. He assured me that my friend was right. Thank God! At least I won't have to bother with the spelling now. Anyway, it isn't anything too serious and can be remedied with some ab-strengthening exercises. Come to think of it, I need some ab-strengthening of my own if I am serious about toning my tummy. One of these days I will get right down to it. Maybe tomorrow ...

S.

Diastasis recti may be a complicated name. But there is an easy way to find out if you have it. Lie down on your back, knees bent, feet placed flat on the ground. Now, as if doing a crunch, lift your head and shoulders above the ground. Place your index and middle finger just below the belly button and you will detect a cavity between two muscles. If this cavity is bigger than the width of your two fingers, you would be diagnosed as having the condition. But why does it happen? So that, sometime during your pregnancy, when you were swelling up to accommodate the growing foetus, the left and the right sides of your abdominal muscles could part a little to create a gap, thereby giving rise to diastasis recti.

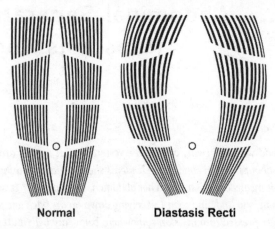

Normal   **Diastasis Recti**

What you need to know:

✓ Abdominal separation is usually triggered during pregnancy (about one-third of all pregnant women are likely to get it), but it may also occur during delivery.

✓ There is no tear in the said muscles; they just spread out so as to grow thinner and more apart.

✓ There is no accompanying pain though the pressure exerted by the foetus may cause backache in pregnant women due to the absence of a firm abdominal support. This pain will ease off after delivery. As such, abdominal separation is less of a concern after delivery than during pregnancy because the internal stress on the abdominals (due to the baby) is no longer exerting a force against them.

How to deal with it:

✓ Post-delivery exercise can help you manage the condition by strengthening your abdomen. Initially, when the gap is wider it is best to stick to Kegels, abdominal compression and pelvic tilts. Avoid exercises that twist your spine for they can worsen the gap.

✓ When the gap shrinks to less than two fingers wide, you can perform the following exercises:

1. **Crunches:** Lie down on an inclined bench (this eases the pressure on your abs), knees bent, hands placed behind your head and your lower back pressed down flat on the bench.

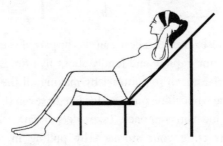

Contract your abs and lift your head and shoulders a few inches, exhaling as you do so. Hold the pose, breathing normally, and then return to the starting position. Do this twelve times.

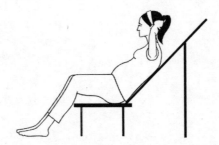

2. **Splinting:** This is a slight variation of the abdominal crunch mentioned above and requires you to wrap a towel around your stomach, with the free ends in front. As you lift your shoulders away from the bench, pull the towel ends towards one another. This action provides extra support to your abdomen.

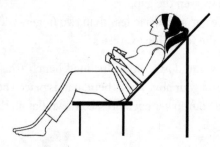

3. **Breathing exercises:** These can also be part of your regimen:
    ☞ Say 'hut' rapidly and loudly about five times. It causes your stomach to contract by making all the air inside come whooshing out. Do this five to seven times a day.
    ☞ Lie down on your back. Take a deep breath, then exhale, contracting your stomach by pulling in your belly button as far as you can towards the spine. Inhale and relax. Do this ten times.

29

Post-Partum Depression

Dear Diary,

Something strange happened to me this afternoon. Mia had just fallen asleep, the household help had come, attended to the chores and gone, and I found myself all alone, with nothing to do. And just like that, tears started rolling down my eyes. Slowly at first and then in a giant torrent. They just wouldn't stop. I didn't know what was happening to me. I kept thinking about my life before pregnancy and how I would never get it back. I felt sorry for myself. And for the mess I was in. And it made me cry even louder. Almost an hour passed before I was able to control my anguish. Even as I think about it now, I feel ashamed of my outburst. I wonder what had come over me.

Yours,
S.

First of all, it is important to distinguish between baby blues and post-partum depression (PPD). Almost all new mothers go through a phase where they feel overwhelmed by what is happening to and around them. It will leave them feeling anxious, miserable and wanting to break down. These are the baby blues and will usually last a couple of weeks. Post-partum depression is real depression involving an inability to get out of the blue funk in which new mothers may find themselves and it requires professional help. Research suggests that 10–15 per cent of new mothers may face post-partum depression. Though serious, the condition is definitely treatable.

What you need to know:

✓ PPD may vary in intensity. Some mothers may suffer from a milder version while others may get completely bogged down by it. New mothers—especially those with schizophrenic or bipolar tendencies—may also be prone to a post-partum psychosis which could possibly drive them to harm themselves or others.

✓ Some believe that hormonal changes are at the root of PPD. Others posit that external factors, such as social pressure to get back to normal as quickly as possible and the lack of helping hands in modern nuclear families to bring up the baby, are more to be blamed.

✓ Typical symptoms include weeping, sleeplessness, overeating or an inability to eat;inability to concentrate; needless anxiety about the baby's health; lack of interest in the baby; being exhausted all the time; feeling sad, hopeless, miserable, frustrated, angry and agitated; getting nightmares and wanting to be or fearing to be alone.

✓ PPD can affect any mother. In some cases, it may make its presence felt during the pregnancy itself. In others, it may show itself a couple of weeks after the delivery rather than immediately after.

✓ Most mothers may not realize that they are suffering from PPD.

✓ Treatment for PPD could include counselling and, in a few

cases, medication. Making positive lifestyle changes too will help.

How to deal with it:

✓ Cut yourself some slack. There is no such thing as a perfect mother and you shouldn't aspire to become one. Setting high standards is stress-inducing and makes you prone to depression when you fail to live up to them.

✓ I have said this before and I will say it again—use all the help you can get. There is no heroism in trying to do everything alone. Hire extra help, delegate chores, get your family members to pitch in with the baby and split night watches with your partner. This will contribute to a more peaceful frame of mind.

✓ I know someone who has a little trick for when she is feeling down. She puts on her brightest lipstick and suddenly the world is a better place. Be like her—put on your best outfit; get your stylist to give you a trendy haircut at home; splash on your favourite perfume; and wear your favourite make-up. It makes a world of a difference, trust me!

✓ Some me-time is essential. Get out of the house once in a while. Shop. Or window-shop. Go to your favourite restaurant. Or catch a movie. Meet up with friends. Or plan a clandestine date with your partner. If you feel guilty about leaving your baby in someone else's care, remind yourself that it is for your—and by extension your baby's—benefit.

✓ Put on your sweats and get moving. Nothing like happy endorphins to bust those blues!

✓ Eat. Low blood sugar may be one reason why you are feeling down in the dumps. A good mood may be just a healthy snack away.

✓ Don't be afraid to show your emotions. If you feel like having a good cry, have one. You will feel better afterwards. If you've been grumpy all day, tune into your favourite sitcom and laugh out loud with the characters. If something is preying on your mind, confide in your partner. Or, as I have said before, vent it all out in your diary.

✓ Having said all this, if the symptoms persist for more than a couple of weeks, seek professional help.

30
Stress

Dear Diary,

I am walking in the woods. Tall, thick trees keep me company and there is just enough sunlight filtering through the leaves to light up my path. I can hear a brook babbling nearby, but I can't see it. I am collecting wildflowers in my basket to carry back home when, suddenly, the trees part and I find myself in a meadow at the foot of snow-covered peaks. A cool wind blows from these mountains and I breathe it in, feeling all my cares melt away into nothing. I feel happy. And at peace... Before you think I have run away from my responsibilities, let me tell you that I am right where I am supposed to be—watching over Mia as she settles into a deep sleep. It's just a technique Namita has advised me to try whenever I am feeling too stressed out. It involves thinking up things that make me happy—in my case, all things close to nature. And you know what? As I escape, emotionally, into the wonderland that my mind conjures up, I can actually feel the stress ebbing away. Suddenly, I am not angry anymore. Or frustrated. Or anxious. Or even tired. Can you believe it?

Picnicking in the woods, yours,
S.

It may sound surprising but stress in limited quantities isn't such a bad thing. It's just the impetus your body needs to cope with the many demands that are made on it. It's when the stress gets out

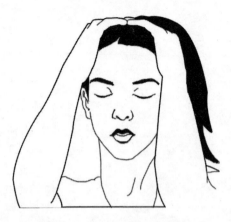

of hand does the problem start. And, as new mothers everywhere will tell you, they face a number of situations day in and day out which can bring this about—sleeplessness; physical discomfort lingering from delivery; a frequently crying baby, a frequently hungry baby; lack of sufficient help, piled-up chores... Sounds like a nightmare? It need not be. As long as you admit that you have a problem and that you are willing to make some changes in your life and get help—whether from friends and family or professionally—this potential nightmare can be transformed once more into the magical time that this period actually is.

What you need to know:

✓ The process of delivery itself is stress-inducing. The levels of epinephrine and cortisol—hormones responsible for inducing psychological stress—rise by a massive 500 per cent during labour.

✓ Post-delivery, the stress is due to external factors—physical pain, changes in routine brought about by the baby, and so on. And also by your own state of mind—expecting too much from yourself and from those around you; unnecessarily fretting about the baby's health; constantly worrying about how you will regain your pre-pregnancy figure; thinking the worst no matter what, and so on. These have physical and psychological effects.

✓ Stress doesn't affect only you; it affects the baby too and not just mood-wise. As I have already mentioned in Section Two, stress hampers the production of oxytocin, a hormone generated in the brain which puts the mammary glands into action and ensures that the milk flows through the ducts and sinuses and reaches your baby. So, high stress could mean less milk for your baby.

How to deal with it:

✓ Identify the causes which are adding to your stress. If they are the kind that you can work on, do so. If lack of help is making you anxious, ask family or friends to come and stay over while you get the hang of playing mother. If you can't turn a blind eye to the dust on the furniture, pay your domestic help extra to clean it. That way, there would be fewer reasons to be stressed about.

✓ There are many things which you must do each day and, sometimes, just thinking of them adds to your stress. So why not make a to-do list every morning starting with the top-priority chores? Tick them off as you deal with them. Just seeing your list grow shorter will add to your sense of ease and keep stress at bay.

✓ In order to ensure that your state of mind isn't adding to your woes, surround yourself with positive energy. Allow sunlight to stream into your home. Stay in touch with people who are supportive and who make you happy. Arrange fresh flowers in vases. Put up pleasing pictures on the walls. All these have a way of infusing positivity in the mind.

✓ Try yoga and meditation. Both are great stress-busters.

✓ Get some sleep. Any situation that seems unmanageable to your sleep-deprived mind will seem less so after a power nap.

✓ Set boundaries. Don't take on additional responsibilities knowing that you won't be able to handle them. The magic word here is, 'No!'

✓ There are ways in which you can coax your body into relaxing. My favourites include:

Tension-relaxation—To relax both mind and body:
Lie down on your back and place one pillow under your head and another under your knees. Your arms are to be at your sides, and the legs, straight and apart. One after the other, tighten each body part and then relax. Do this in the following sequence:

i.   Make a fist and tighten your hands. Relax.

ii.   Bring your arms up, bend them at the elbow and, keeping your palms open, tighten the arms and forearms. Relax.

iii. Pull your shoulders up close to your ears, tighten and then relax.

iv.   Flex your ankles and clench your thigh muscles. Relax.

v.   Clench your buttocks together. Relax.

vi.   Stiffen your head and neck, and then release the tension.

vii. Clench your jaws and mouth, scrounge up your eyes, and wrinkle your forehead and then relax.

viii. Breathe deeply five times. Feel the stress melt each time you exhale. Replace it with positive affirmations: I am calm. I am relaxed. I am stress-free.

Abdominal/Diaphragmatic Breathing—To induce calm and quiet:
Sit comfortably on a chair. Place your hands on your stomach, breathe in and out. Feel your stomach go out when you breathe in, feel it come in when you breathe out. The chest and the shoulders must remain in place. Do this slowly and try to make every breath last longer than the one before it. Do this for three to four minutes daily.

Imagery—To flood your mind with happy thoughts:
It's like dreaming, except that you are awake. Lie down on your side, bend your knees and place a pillow under your head. Now that you are comfortable, close your eyes and dream up things that make you happy. Srishti always imagines herself surrounded by nature: snow-covered mountains, green meadows, rain, forests, and so on. The more detail she adds to her landscape—the crunch of snow under her feet, the gurgle of a brook, the dappled sunlight streaming through tall, thick trees—the more involved her mind gets in creating those images. And when one's mind is busy churning out happy images, where is the time to dwell on stressful situations?

Tip: Choose a room that is quiet, cosy and free of distractions when practising these techniques.

✓ If your stress gets out of hand and you feel absolutely burned out, don't hesitate to seek professional help in the form of psychotherapy and counselling.

31
Backache

Dear Diary,

Oh, this backache! I am sick of it. Not one movement can I make without being aware of just how bad it is. I know I should have expected this considering I have always had a weak back. Having a job that requires you to spend all your time hunched over a computer on your desk can't be easy on the spine. Tottering about with a protruding stomach during pregnancy must have been equally bad. But while I could once afford to spend a couple of weeks in bed to give it time to recover, I can't do that anymore, not with so many other things that are vying for my attention. And so I believe I must carry on valiantly...

In pain, yours,
S.

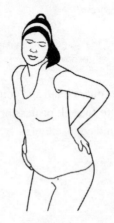

New mothers are no strangers to backaches. In fact, most would consider it a constant companion—unwanted but one that must be put up with. But even this pesky guest can't linger forever. For most women, the condition gets resolved in a few months. For those like Srishti who suffered from it even before pregnancy, it may take slightly longer. The key to a faster recovery, I tell my clients, is a good diet, correct posture and mild exercise.

What you need to know:

✓ Most women are introduced to backache during pregnancy. As your tummy expands forward, you tend to lean backward to maintain your centre of gravity. The extra pressure which it puts on your lower back can cause backache which could linger well after delivery.

✓ Pregnancy and delivery involve many physical and hormonal changes in your body which leave your joints and back weak and vulnerable. It is best to take things slow and steady, and to ration your movements until your body gets a chance to recover its strength.

✓ Heavy breasts too may contribute to the problem.

✓ If you aren't paying attention to your posture when feeding, changing or carrying your baby, you could worsen the backache.

How to deal with it:

✓ Ensure correct posture no matter what you are doing (Refer to Chapter Six in this section for more details.).

✓ Both sitting and standing for long hours put stress on your back. From time to time, take a break. If you've been on your feet for a while, pull up a chair and put your feet up, literally! Likewise, if you've been working at your desk for hours together, take a walk and use the time to stretch your back.

✓ Stow away your heels for a while. They aren't worth the backache.

✓ Avoid lifting heavy objects, except for the baby, at least for the first eight weeks. This is one time you should consider putting others to work for you.

✓ Consider using a harness or a sling for carrying your baby.

✓ All the weight you had put on during pregnancy puts additional pressure on your back. As soon as possible and permissible, get started on an exercise regimen to knock it off.

✓ This may sound like a tall order but try and get as much rest as possible. Give your back the pampering it deserves—hot baths, hot-water bags, soothing massages, and so on.

✓ In addition to this, I would like to show you a few stretching exercises that provide relief from backache. Perform them for about five to ten minutes daily for best results.

Note: Do consult your doctor before launching into an exercise regimen to ensure it does not aggravate the backache.

Stretching exercises

These will make a significant difference in your flexibility and strength, and alleviate your backache. They can be performed as frequently as needed throughout the day.

1a. **Pelvic Tilt—Standing**
   See exercise on p. 127.
1b. **Pelvic Tilt—Lying Down**
   Lie on your back on a mat with knees bent; tilt your pelvis

by drawing the tailbone up and pressing down the back, pulling in the abdominal muscles. Hold the position for five to ten seconds, release and repeat for seven counts.

2. **Cat-Camel Stretch**
   See exercise on p. 133.

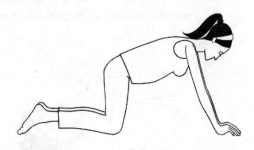

Slowly arch your back upwards (like the hump of a camel), tucking the tailbone under. Again hold for five seconds. Repeat both movements seven times.

3. **Spinal Flexion—Seated**

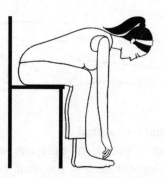

Sit on a chair with your feet side by side on the floor. Move the knees apart, bend forward, allowing your abdomen to rest between your legs. Hold for five to ten seconds and repeat seven times.

4. **Knee to Chest—Lying Down**

   a. **Double Knee:** Lie on your back, knees bent and feet together. Reach out to the back of your thighs and pull the knees towards your chest. Repeat five times.

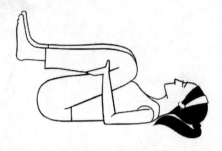

   b. **Single Knee:** Lie on your back, bend one knee and pull it towards the outer side of your chest. Change legs. Repeat five times.

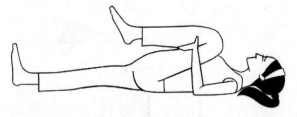

5a. **Spinal Rotation—Seated**

   Sit on a chair, stretch the right arm across your belly and grasp the opposite side of the chair. Look over your right shoulder, twisting your lower back and mid-back. Repeat on each side for three counts.

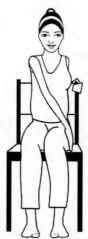

5b. Spinal Rotation—Lying Down

Lie on your back, placing your hands under your head. Bend your legs at the knees, keeping them close together. Drop both bent legs to your right side and turn your head to the left. Hold for five seconds. Feel the lower back muscles relax and lengthen. Then, keeping your knees together, turn to the centre, drop them to your left side, turning your head to the right. Repeat for three counts.

32

Bad Posture

Dear Diary,

I've just had a breakthrough, thanks to Namita. Realizing that my back was hurting very badly, she taught me a few exercises to relieve the pain. And you know what? The results are beginning to show. She also taught me how important it is to maintain a good posture. You'd think a grown-up woman like me would know how to stand and sit. But when I went through the paces with her, I saw that I was getting even those basics wrong. On her advice, I have lately taken to watching myself in a mirror whenever I can. Just so that I know I am standing up straight and sitting down right. It seems a little vain, but I guess it is necessary. And it's working. She has also passed on posture suggestions for when I am with the baby. Is it time for me to finally say bye-bye to poor posture? I sure hope so.

S.

I truly believe that the one thing you can work on as soon as you are up and about is your posture. Posture is important no matter which activity you are engaging in—from standing up, sitting down and sleeping to carrying, feeding and changing your baby. These last few, especially, are new movements for you and since you are going to be repeating them for quite some time now, it makes sense to learn how to do them correctly right

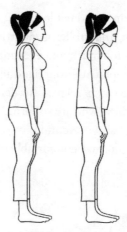

from the start. By paying just a little attention to the way you carry yourself, you can prevent your already-taxed joints and back from getting further traumatized, and thereby aid their complete recovery.

What you need to know:

✓ Good posture protects your body from injuries. Bad posture puts strain on your joints, bones and muscles.

✓ An ideal posture is neutral in the sense that it follows the natural curvature of your spine, thus putting the least strain on it.

✓ Good posture is easy to maintain if your abs and upper back are strong.

How to deal with it:

Practise getting into the right posture for the following activities:

✓ **Walking a stroller**

    i.   Keep your head and chin up, your shoulders down and your chest out.

ii. Bend your arms but don't lock your elbows.

iii. While pushing the stroller, avoid straining your wrists by flexing them too much and exerting pressure on them. Instead, attempt to use your hand and shoulder strength and keep the wrists relaxed (in neutral position). This will benefit those who are suffering from swollen wrists on account of water retention.

iv. Stick to your normal, comfortable stride.

Fitness Tip: Choose a stroller according to your height.

✓ **Carrying the baby**

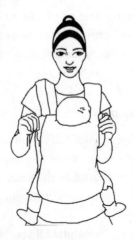

i. Keep your spine straight, not hunched, not bent backward or forward.

ii. It is always a good idea to centre your baby to your body. Carrying him on any one side will affect your centre of gravity.

iii. Once again, keep your wrist relaxed as you hold the baby.

✓ **Changing the baby's diaper**
  i.   Make sure your work surface is a little above elbow level. This will avoid your bending forward and rounding your back to change the diaper.
  ii. Keep the supplies handy, not somewhere that requires you to bend or twist.

✓ **Nursing the baby**
  Refer to Section Two, Chapter One for different positions for breastfeeding.

✓ **Standing up**
  i.   Relax your shoulders.
  ii. Keep your spine tall and in the neutral position. Your head and neck should be aligned with it.
  iii. Lift your chest and pull in your abdomen.
  iv. Distribute your weight equally on both feet.

✓ **Sitting down**
  i.   Use a chair with a straight back and an arm support.
  ii. Provide additional support to your lower back by tucking in a small, firm pillow.
  iii. Have a low stool handy to rest your feet on.

✓ **Lifting heavy objects**
  i.   If you *must* lift them, stand with your feet apart.
  ii. Bend at your knees rather than your waist.
  iii. Keep your back straight.
  iv. Use your arms and legs rather than your back to lift the object.
  v.   If carrying groceries, divide your shopping equally in two bags and carry them on both arms.

✓ **Sleeping**

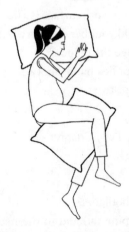

i.   Use a firm mattress, one that is not too soft, nor too hard.
ii. Sleep on your side with a pillow between your legs. If you tend to sleep on your back, bend your knees and tuck a pillow below them to support your back.

✓ **Getting out of bed**

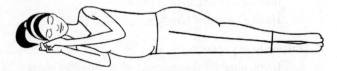

i.   Turn on one side, shoulders, hips, knees, and legs together to prevent twisting.
ii. Swing your legs over the side of the bed and to the ground and use them to push your body into a sitting position.
iii. Protect your sore abs with your hands to ensure there is no jerking.

iv. To get into bed, support your abs with your hands as you sit down, as close to the head of the bed as possible. Swing your legs onto the bed, one after the other and lie down gently.

Take it from me: It is easy to make a mountain out of a molehill, especially when you have a baby to take care of, but none of these concerns should cause you needless worry. If you know how to deal with them (and, based on my many experiences of working with new mothers, I've tried to share that with you), it is possible to deal with them all. The mantra I would like you to take away from this section is, 'Divide and conquer'. Divide responsibilities between you and your family so that you can conquer the many-headed, multi-tasking monster that is parenthood. It will give you some time of your own to rest and get rejuvenated, and to help you look forward to this period with great joy and anticipation.

SECTION SIX

WELL-BEING

A couple of months after delivery, several other issues begin to demand your attention. Those of you who have put your job on hold may have to return to work, so that you now have to juggle your career, the home *and* the baby. It is enough to make you feel overused and overwrought—a state of mind that is sure to make you ignore your diet and reach out for some fattening comfort food. That is why it is important that you learn to spend some time every day looking after yourself. If you can keep stress away, you can keep temptation at bay. This section deals with miscellaneous matters—how to pamper yourself; how to keep your mind focused and resolved on losing weight; and how to plan your return to work. I have also included a chapter that is really meant for your partner—it explains the role he can play in making your life slightly easier. In brief, with this section, I hope to inculcate in you a sense of well-being which will go a long way in helping you do justice to all your different roles.

33
Spoil Yourself Silly

Dear Diary,

I have a confession to make. I have become a massage addict. I tried it for the first time in my second month after delivery and let me tell you, it was bliss. There is nothing more relaxing than the act of surrendering your body to the ministrations of an expert masseuse. The good part is that I don't even have to step outside my home to receive it. My friend recommended a maalishwaali who comes home to give massages. And boy, is she good! She knows just the right moves to ease the tension from your muscles. Gently. But firmly. My body is like putty in her hands and I feel relaxed and oh-so-pampered after a session with her. I have had a couple of massages since and intend on scheduling more of them. And why not? To borrow a catchphrase, I am worth it.

S.

If your mind is going round in circles juggling home, work, baby and your diet, and you feel like you are being sucked into a whirlpool from which there is no escape, it can mean only one thing. You need a break. A break from routine. A vacation may be ideal but not practical, given the circumstances. So consider shorter breaks—from a few minutes to a couple of hours—taken every day, just so that you can stay in touch with yourself. Rest.

Relax. Rejuvenate. Before plunging headlong, once more, into your hectic routine.

What you need to know:

Giving birth to a baby and raising him or her sorely tests both body and mind. The only way to put them both at ease is to find the time to spoil yourself silly. Trust me, you deserve it.

How to deal with it:

✓ **Make an appointment at a spa.** Say spa and you think of soft music, low lighting, packs and wraps, gentle massages ... what better way to relax than this? All you need to do is surrender both mind and body and let the experts work their magic. You could consider different options:

   i.   Massage: It reduces anxiety, alleviates depression and relieves muscle aches and pains. It even induces sound sleep.

   ii. Reflexology: It involves applying pressure to specific areas of the hands, feet and ears. This allows energy to flow freely through your body, increases the blood flow to a corresponding part of your body, and promotes toxin removal.

   iii. Hydrotherapy: The therapeutic use of warm water, usually in a whirlpool tub, is used in many hospitals and birthing centres to induce relaxation.

✓ **Try and catch up on sleep.** It is the easiest, the most effective stress-buster there can be. Of course, you will have to try and match your baby's timings with your own. Sleep when he sleeps. Or get someone in your family to supervise the baby in order to allow you to catch up on your own forty winks. If sleep eludes you despite your best intentions, try the following tricks:

i. Don't exercise close to bedtime; it might wind you up instead of down.

ii. Try and give your mind some rest. An overactive mind isn't conducive to sleep.

iii. Too many trips to the bathroom interrupting your sleep? Limit fluid intake after eight p.m. Fulfil your daily quota of water before then.

iv. This might seem a difficult proposition, but try and get to bed when you're tired. If you wait until you are overtired, sleep may actually elude you.

✓ **Get a sauna or a steam bath.** It helps eliminate accumulated toxins through sweat, promotes circulation, and creates a sense of relaxation.

Post-Partum Massage

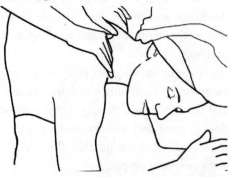

A post-partum massage may be just the thing which your weary body and mind need to cope with the stresses of pregnancy and delivery. It is particularly helpful in relieving muscular aches and pains that afflict new mothers, especially pain in the back, the arms and the shoulders brought on by breastfeeding; it also helps eliminate medicinal and toxic wastes from your body.

Whether you choose light massages or deeper, more intensive techniques, an expert masseuse can also help improve postural imbalances and break down adhesions that may have formed as a result of surgery. Some other benefits include:

- ☞ Sound sleep: Studies indicate that massage therapy boosts the delta brain waves which are associated with deep sleep. If you sleep soundly, you will automatically feel well rested. And here's an interesting fact: sound sleep helps improve your metabolism. That, coupled with the right diet and exercise, can speed up fat loss.

- ☞ Rest and relaxation: Massage therapy helps ease the tension from your muscles, promote circulation, and lower stress hormones. The feeling is one of total relaxation.

- ☞ Better hormonal balance: It is believed that massage therapy can reduce the level of stress hormone cortisol in your body. It also regulates the presence of dopamine and serotonin (associated with depression), and norepinephrine (associated with cardiovascular problems).

- ☞ Decrease in swelling: By promoting circulation in the body and by hastening the elimination of toxic wastes and fluids, massage therapy helps your body regain its fluid balance and reduces swelling. The right massage moves will also ensure that the water in your body settles in the right places.

- ☞ Better breastfeeding: Massage therapy may help relax chest muscles and increase levels of prolactin, a hormone associated with lactation, there by helping breastfeeding.

34

Mind Games

Dear Diary,

I used to think losing weight was a physical activity. Eating right, working up a sweat through exercise... But, as Namita puts it, the real inspiration for it comes from within: the mind. The mind is a wonderful thing. If it takes a stand, no mountain is too high and no weight loss target too difficult. And so, she advises, I must concentrate on making an ally of my mind. If I do that, good results will follow automatically.

S.

To repeat what Srishti mentions in her diary, losing weight is as much a psychological as a physical game, especially when your

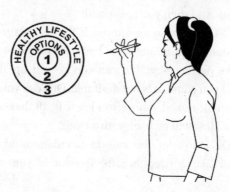

mind is distracted by your various responsibilities. A stressed mind is a liability, a weakness that can impact your weight loss goals. Here are a few strategies for better mind control.

What you need to know:

If you make up your mind, nothing can stop you from reaching your goal.

How to deal with it:

✓ **WANT.** If you don't want something, you will never really strive for it. As a child, you behaved exactly as your parents wished just so you could get that toy you wanted. This is no different. If you want to lose weight just as badly as you wanted that toy, you will go to great lengths to achieve it— control your cravings; stay true to your eating plan; limit sweets, fried, oily and creamy foods; and work up a good sweat with exercise.

✓ **BELIEVE.** Believe that you can lose weight. Believe that you have the willpower to do so. Negative thinking never helped anybody. If you don't believe in yourself, why should the rest of us? Face the battle of the bulge believing that you *will* win. And then you really will!

✓ **BALANCE:** Choose an approach that is balanced and can be sustained on a long-term basis. A crash diet may sound like the perfect plan, but can you keep it up all your life? Even if you could, it is not desirable. One day you will give in to temptation and, before you know it, all that extra weight you had lost will be back with a bang!

✓ **RELAX.** Don't let the calorie calculations wind you up. Relax. Take a deep breath. De-clutter you mind of all negative emotions. Then start afresh. With a clean slate and a stress-free mind.

✓ **PERSEVERE.** It is easy to be motivated in short bursts but to sustain it for life ... now, that takes effort. So try and think of more than one reason to lose weight—it will make you healthy; it will make you look good; you will feel more confident; your friends will compliment you and want to be like you. These will keep you going even when you are short on motivation. Also, find something to do which you enjoy. If you enjoy your workout, you are less likely to skip it. It doesn't take too long for a day's holiday to turn into a much-longer vacation from diet and exercise. So, keep at it.

35

Getting Back to Work

Dear Diary,

I consider it a blessing that I don't have a conventional job. I can work from home and being a freelancer means that I can pick and choose my assignments. Imagine if I had to report to work once I had used up my maternity leave! To get back to the demanding schedules, the impossible deadlines, the stress—all inevitable fallouts of a successful career these days. Half my time would have been spent worrying about Mia. Had she been fed on time? Was she crying? Was she missing me? At home, I would have been worrying about work. At work, I would have been worrying about home. In the end, I think I wouldn't have done justice to either. I wonder how other women manage it.

S.

Srishti is bang on when she visualizes just what sort of problems working mothers are likely to face. And while she herself was spared the burden of returning to a full-time job soon after delivery, you may not be equally lucky. In this case, I have just the suggestions to help you juggle your tasks more efficiently.

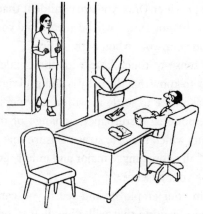

BACK TO WORK!

What you need to know:

Returning to work after maternity leave won't be child's play. On the one hand, it may trouble you to spend time away from your baby, and you may find yourself obsessing over what he is doing in your absence. On the other hand, you may find it difficult to get back to the pressures of work—especially the long hours, the short deadlines and other work-related problems. Along with all this, you may find it hard to continue breastfeeding your baby.

How to deal with it:

✓   First and foremost, don't feel guilty about returning to work. Just because you are itching to get back doesn't mean that you love your baby less or that you are a bad mother.

✓   Make arrangements for reliable childcare. Do a thorough background check before entrusting your baby with a childcare provider. Once you are confident that your choice is trustworthy, your mind will be at ease and you will be able to focus on your work when in the office.

✓ It makes sense to touch base with the childcare provider once a day to know that the baby is doing all right. Your baby too will take time to settle in with a new person, so check for any emotional disturbances, change of diet or bowel movements which indicate stress. Ensure that you are kept abreast of all happenings—major and minor—in your baby's life during your absence.

✓ Confide in your employer and see if you can work out a slightly easy routine that will allow you to ease into your work. Ask if you can work from home or avail of flexible timings.

✓ Put your time management skills to use. Have a to-do list at the start of each day. It will help you prioritize home and office tasks according to their importance. The least important ones can wait or, if necessary, be skipped if you run out of time.

✓ Always have a Plan B in place. If the childcare provider needs to take the day off, have a few members in your family shortlisted to take her place at short notice. Either you or your partner should be prepared to come home early in case there is a medical emergency.

✓ If you intend to continue breastfeeding, make arrangements to have your child fed during breaks at work or make it a point to pump milk on your day off so that it can be used when you are away.

✓ As I keep saying, don't try to manage it all by yourself. Get your partner and the rest of your family involved in taking care of the baby.

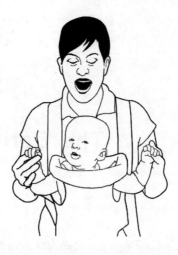

Do spare some time to attend to your own well-being. Try to do things you love—listening to music, reading a book—to help you relax and take your mind off your problems.

36

The Caring Dad

Dear Diary,

My husband and I had a fight last night. He argued that I no longer had any time for him. And I complained that he never volunteered to take care of the baby. I guess we both have a point. Since he works long hours (and is usually too tired to stay up nights with the baby), I end up looking after the baby on my own. I resent it a little bit—that he gets to go out and have his own life while I am stuck with changing diapers and cleaning up. No wonder evenings find me grumpy and grouchy and hardly in the mood to spend quality time with him. It has created this great big divide between the two of us and I just don't know how to overcome it.

S.

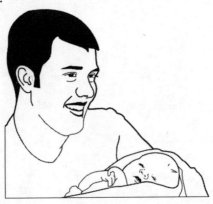

This chapter is really for you, Dad! If you feel that you have gained a baby but lost your wife and you are no more than a spectator in their lives, here's what you can do to change things for the better.

What you need to know:

✓ Your partner's sex drive may suffer due to hormonal changes brought about by pregnancy and delivery. Poor body image after pregnancy too may affect intimacy. Plus, having to take care of the baby all day long means she is tired and distracted, and sex may be the last thing on her mind.

✓ Time becomes a precious commodity, and your partner may find her hands too full to pay any attention to you.

✓ She may feel flustered, she may experience mood swings, and feel unloved and unappreciated at this time.

How to deal with it:

✓ Wait for at least six weeks before initiating the idea of sex. This will give her body enough time to recover from the delivery. Try and dispel her fears about not looking her best. Compliment her, woo her with flowers, take her out on a date ... it will make her feel wanted and appreciated. If pain during sex is an issue, talk it out with her. Discuss positions that will take the pressure off her abdomen. It is best to take things slowly initially.

✓ Instead of feeling jealous, why not give your partner a helping hand? Take on tasks, like changing the baby's diaper and giving him a bath. Talk with him, take him out on walks, rock him to sleep. It will help you bond with the baby and make you feel more involved in his life. It will also give your partner some precious me-time and time to focus on both of you as well.

✓ It is important to extend your support to your partner at all times. Not only baby work, but do take on some of the household responsibilities as well. Communication is the key. Talk with her, understand her problems, help out with the solutions and generally make her feel like she is not alone in all this.

37
FAQ

Dear Diary,

More questions. They never stop, do they? It's a good thing Namita is always only a phone call away. Makes it easier to seek answers to all my doubts.

S.

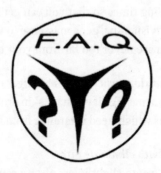

1. **How soon after delivery can I get a massage?**

   If there were no complications, you can get one as soon as you are comfortable. If there were, it is best to seek your doctor's advice. Try and get in at least three to five massages in the first six months. Ensure your masseuse is an expert in post-partum massages and discuss comfortable positions with her to derive maximum benefit. For instance, some women may like to be facedown, others may prefer to lie on their sides to take the pressure off their breasts.

2. *What if I have had a Caesarean?*
Then, it is best to wait for a week or two before you consider getting a massage. In any case, consult your doctor about it. Instruct your masseuse to stay away from your abdomen and the surgical scar. After about five to six weeks have elapsed, your abdomen can be massaged gently. An added bonus: this will help the wound to heal and the scar to fade.

3. *But where is the time for such indulgence?*
You will find time only if you provide for it. The simplest way is to get your family to pitch in and supervise the baby while you get your massage. Try and schedule one in between feeding times so that you can get away for a while. If you cannot visit a spa, get a masseuse to visit you at home. That way you are never too far from your baby.

4. *Are there conditions where such massages can be harmful?*
Avoid getting a massage if you have skin problems or medical complications which need clearance from a physician.

5. *Can a steam bath eliminate fat?*
No. You may weigh slightly less after a sauna bath but that is only due to a continuous loss of water from the body through perspiration. As soon as you replenish it through food and water, you will revert to your original weight.

6. *Is a steam bath the same as a sauna?*
No. A steam bath induces sweat by generating and circulating steam. It creates high humidity, and the temperature

generated is much lower than the sauna, about 40° C. Sauna induces sweat by circulating dry heat in a cubicle for a specific time period. Here, temperatures can reach up to 60°C. People with respiratory problems might find this low-humidity environment uncomfortable.

Take it from me: You will manage work. You will manage home. You will manage your baby. *And* you will manage your diet and exercise plan. Everything will work out if you have just one weapon in your arsenal: *motivation*. If you are motivated, you can move mountains. Of course, motivation won't just happen. You will have to work on it every day of your life. My advice? Take one day at a time and the rest of your life will automatically fall into place.

A Final Word

In their hearts, everybody knows what they must do to lose weight—eat less, exercise more often. So why do they need books? Because they are looking for a helping hand. A friend with stories who they can identify and from whom they can get inspiration. A guide who will dole out helpful tips. A philosopher who will give them hope. I have tried to make this book all that, and more. And I have, I hope, thrown a life jacket of sorts to new mothers who feel as if they are swimming against the tide. If they consider it as such, then I will think this a job well done.

Acknowledgements

This book has come to fruition thanks to the concerted efforts of an entire team. Without their encouragement and support, this book would not have been possible.

I am extremely grateful to my publishers, HarperCollins India, for giving me the opportunity to present the concept for my book, *Post-Baby Bounce*. They have guided me towards producing what I consider an exceptional book that will hopefully serve as an invaluable guide for all those who wish to reach their target weight.

My thanks to my editors, Neelini Sarkar and Debasri Rakshit, who offered valuable insights and suggestions during the entire process.

I wish to acknowledge the inputs of my creative consultant, Runa Jog, for helping me with the preliminary edits, including the case studies, and for assisting me in laying out the text in a reader-friendly format.

Finally, I wish to thank my clients for sharing with me their real-life stories and experiences which gave me the inspiration and the impetus to write this book.